respond, how the experience affects their lives, how they use or fail to use available services, and ultimately, how the system fails them. The authors show how current hospital or clinic care—which traditionally has treated only the acute stages of an illness—has neglected the complex social, psychological, physical, and financial needs of the chronically ill.

Strauss and Corbin offer new ways of viewing long-term illness, stressing the lifelong treatment required, outlining the several phases of chronic illness, and most importantly focusing on the overall quality of the patient's life. They make recommendations—such as integrating home care with hospital care—that will address the wide-ranging needs of the chronically ill.

THE AUTHORS

ANSELM STRAUSS is a professor emeritus of sociology, University of California, San Francisco. His numerous books include *Time for Dying* (with B. Glaser) and *The Politics of Pain Management* (with S. Fagerhaugh), among others. JULIET M. CORBIN is a lecturer in the Department of Nursing, San Jose State University. She has worked as a nurse both in a hospital and in the homes of the chronically ill. Strauss and Corbin are coauthors of *Unending Work and Care* (Jossey-Bass, 1988).

D0812411

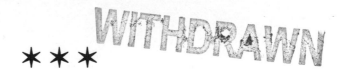
Shaping a New
Health Care System

Anselm Strauss
Juliet M. Corbin

Shaping a New
Health Care System

*The Explosion
of Chronic Illness
as a Catalyst for Change*

Jossey-Bass Publishers
San Francisco   •   London   •   1988

SHAPING A NEW HEALTH CARE SYSTEM
The Explosion of Chronic Illness as a Catalyst for Change
by Anselm Strauss and Juliet M. Corbin

Copyright © 1988 by: Jossey-Bass Inc., Publishers
350 Sansome Street
San Francisco, California 94104
&
Jossey-Bass Limited
28 Banner Street
London EC1Y 8QE

Library of Congress Cataloging-in-Publication Data

Strauss, Anselm L.
 Shaping a new health care system.

 (Jossey-Bass health series) (Jossey-Bass social
and behavioral science series) (Jossey-Bass public
administration series)
  Bibliography: p.
  Includes index.
  1. Chronically ill—Care—United States.
2. Medical policy—United States. I. Corbin,
Juliet M., date. II. Title. III. Series.
IV. Series: Jossey-Bass social and behavioral
science series.
RA644.5.S76 1988   362.1'0973   88-42801
ISBN 1-55542-116-4

Manufactured in the United States of America

The paper in this book meets the guidelines for
permanence and durability of the Committee on
Production Guidelines for Book Longevity of the
Council on Library Resources.

JACKET DESIGN BY WILLI BAUM

FIRST EDITION

Code 8843

A *joint publication in*

The Jossey-Bass Health Series

The Jossey-Bass
Social and Behavioral Science Series

and

The Jossey-Bass
Public Administration Series

Contents

Preface

Chronic illness poses a major policy issue: How can we deal with the manifestations and effects of this presently incurable and prevalent form of illness? The traditional answer to this issue is to provide efficient clinical interventions and treatments, and the U.S. health care system is based almost exclusively on this clinical orientation. Recently, however, a number of critics have pointed out deficiencies in our health care system, including its apparent lack of support for home health care, financial aid, and counseling for the ill and their families. In *Shaping a New Health Care System,* we address this central issue—surely one of the most pressing of our times—with a more radical stance than is usual. We will argue and demonstrate that the broader implications of chronic illness have never been understood. We do not claim to fully grasp them ourselves, but this book should surely add to the rapidly growing public and professional awareness that the prevalence of chronic illness necessitates profound changes in our health care system and our society itself.

Our own view of health policy issues has been shaped by years of intensive research into the care of the chronically ill, as it is carried out in hospitals and the private homes of the ill. As a result, we have reached a position that rests on a new theoretical framework for the management of chronic illness. We believe this framework can be useful to all the people most intimately involved in caring for the chronically ill: health care practitioners (physicians, nurses, social workers, psychologists, family counselors, home health care practitioners); "policy thinkers" (economists, political scientists, sociologists, policy-

oriented physicians); policy planners and legislators; foundation personnel who are especially interested in health policy;
and, of course, the ill and their families.

Generally, there are three main stages in the implementation of any major change in policy or practice. Stage one includes arguments for and demonstrations of the need for change;
stage two involves determining the general outline of a new,
operative system; and stage three is composed of designing and
implementing the specific aspects of the new system. This book
addresses the first stage directly and the second stage more
generally, although, we hope, with enough specificity to affect
the traditional acute-care approach to chronic illness.

We anchor our arguments in reality by using excerpts
from interviews to show how the chronically ill and their families
experience chronic illness and respond to its effect on their lives,
how and why they use or do not use the health care system,
and how that system helps or fails them. Hence, except for five
introductory chapters and the two final chapters, this book is
composed largely of illustrative quotations from our interviews
with chronically ill people and their marital partners or caretakers. These quotations are supplemented by policy-oriented
commentaries concerning the issues mentioned above and some
additional data from other researchers.

Overview of the Contents

In Part One we introduce the reader to chronic illness,
the U.S. health care system's approach to chronic illness, and
the need for the system's major reform. We also provide a conceptual model of the experiences of the chronically ill. In Chapter
One we briefly introduce our perspective on the implications
of chronic illness for the U.S. health care system. In Chapter
Two we address the prevalence and complex nature of chronic
illness, and in Chapter Three we summarize some of the major
responses of the health care system to the increase in chronic
illness. We discuss the weaknesses of the conventional acute-
care approach to chronic illness in Chapter Four, noting the
various criticisms that have been made of it and the critics'

suggestions for how long-term illnesses and disabilities could be managed. We also point out how we agree and disagree with the critics.

In Part Two we illustrate how the ill and their marital partners experience chronic illness and its management. These experiences have implications for health care policy, some of which are pointed out in the accompanying commentaries. Chapter Five is central to this book, for in it we offer our new theoretical framework for dealing with chronic illness and its increasing influence on the U.S. health care system and policies. In Chapters Six through Nine we describe four distinctly different stages of chronic illness: comeback phases, stable phases, unstable phases, and deterioration. In each chapter we present case illustrations and commentaries on relevant policy.

In Part Three we summarize the implications for health care practice and policy that can be derived from the case illustrations provided in Part Two. In Chapter Ten we detail some of the possible effects on health care practitioners of adopting our framework. And in Chapter Eleven we summarize our conceptual model and present some of the major policy implications of our perspective.

Acknowledgments

We welcome the opportunity to thank the people who read drafts of the manuscript for this book, helped us formulate our ideas about health policy, and contributed to the research that underlies our policy suggestions. Gay Becker and Laura Reif of the University of California, San Francisco, and Peter Conrad of Brandeis University offered helpful critiques of the first draft. Patricia Hess of San Francisco State University and Nancy Horner, a nursing student at San Jose State University, did the same for the final draft. Among the many people who have furthered our ideas or joined us in research on chronic illness have been the late Rue Bucher, University of Illinois; Wolfram Fischer, University of Giessen, West Germany; Berenice Fisher, New York University; Elihu Gerson, Tremont Research Institute, San Francisco; Barney Glaser and Leonard Schatzman,

University of California, San Francisco; Fritz Schuetze, University of Kassel, West Germany; and Leigh Star, University of California, Irvine.

We want to express special appreciation for three research colleagues, all of the University of California, San Francisco, with whom we have recently published volumes on chronic illness: Shizuko Fagerhaugh, Barbara Suczek, and Carolyn Wiener. We also wish to thank Celia Orona and Dorothy Rice of the University of California, San Francisco, for providing data pertaining to chronic illness and helpful references on statistics, respectively.

We thank Lloyd Gross and Laurens White, two San Francisco physicians who referred chronically ill patients to us; Irving Horowitz, editor and publisher of *Society,* who gave us the opportunity to publish some of the policy conclusions now expressed in the last chapter of this book; and the Visiting Nurses of San Francisco and Veterans Administration Medical Center in Palo Alto, California, for allowing us to interview their patients.

Two anonymous reviewers of the original manuscript, commissioned by Jossey-Bass, contributed to a better final draft, as did Fran Strauss, who was of great help in typing the manuscript; William Henry; Alis Temerin; and our copyeditor, Stella Hackell. Most of all we are indebted to the chronically ill people and their "significant others" who shared their experiences of living with and managing chronic illness with us. Some of them can be heard speaking in this book, and we hope their messages will be acted upon by health care practitioners and policymakers.

San Francisco   Anselm Strauss
July 1988   Juliet M. Corbin

The Authors

Anselm Strauss is professor emeritus of sociology, University of California, San Francisco. He received his B.S. degree in biology (1939) from the University of Virginia, and his M.A. and Ph.D. degrees in sociology (1942 and 1945) from the University of Chicago.

Strauss's main research activities have been in medical sociology of work/professions. His research program in medical sociology goes back over two decades and includes studies on dying in hospitals, the management of pain in hospitals, the impact of medical technology on the care of hospitalized patients, and the problems of living with chronic illness. In 1981 he received the Distinguished Medical Sociologist of the Year award from the Medical Sociology section of the American Sociological Association. He received the Cooley Award (1980) and Mead Award (1985) from the Society for the Study of Symbolic Interaction, and was named the 30th Annual Research Scholar of the Year of the University of California, San Francisco (1987). Strauss is a fellow of the American Association for the Advancement of Science (1980). His publications include *Psychiatric Ideologies and Institutions* (1964, with others), *Awareness of Dying* (1965, with B. Glaser), *The Discovery of Grounded Theory* (1967, with B. Glaser), *Time for Dying* (1968, with B. Glaser), *The Politics of Pain Management* (1977, with S. Fagerhaugh), *Chronic Illness and the Quality of Life* (2nd. ed.) (1984, with others), *The Social Organization of Medical Work* (1984, with others), *Qualitative Analysis* (1987), *Hazards in Hospital Care* (1987, with others), and *Unending Work and Care* (1988, with J. Corbin).

He has been a visiting professor at the University of Cambridge (England), the University of Paris, the University of Manchester, the University of Constance, the University of Adelaide, and the University of Hagen.

Juliet M. Corbin is a lecturer in the Department of Nursing, San Jose State University, and a research associate in the Department of Social and Behavioral Sciences, University of California, San Francisco. She received her B.S.N. degree (1963) from Arizona State University, her M.S.N. degree (1972) from San Jose State University, and her D.N.S. degree (1981) from the University of California, San Francisco.

Corbin has taught courses on research and on chronic illness, and she has served as a consultant in these same areas. Her research has focused on chronic illness and the sociology of work. Currently she is studying the integrative role of head nurses and nurse managers who work on medical wards at a Veterans Administration hospital. She has had considerable experience as a nurse, working both in hospitals and, more recently, in the homes of the chronically ill. She has also been a postdoctoral research fellow in the Department of Social and Behavioral Sciences, University of San Francisco.

Corbin has authored or coauthored several research articles and chapters in edited collections and recently coauthored *Unending Work and Care* (1988, with A. Strauss).

Shaping a New
Health Care System

ONE

∗ ∗ ∗ ∗ ∗

How Chronic Illness Is Challenging Our Health Care System

In Part One, we will discuss the importance of chronic illness in the lives of Americans and the role it can play in reshaping the American health care system. Nevertheless, an acute care approach still dominates our system and, thereby, leads to many inadequacies in providing health care for the chronically ill. In Chapter One we outline our general perspective on the major importance of chronic illness for rethinking the nation's health care system. The similarities and differences between our position and that of other critics of the current health care system are suggested.

In Chapter Two, we note that chronic illness is now the prevalent form of illness and has greatly affected health care and facilities. Nevertheless, some of the more far-reaching implications of this prevalence have not yet been recognized. Major characteristics of chronic illness are described and some impacts of the prevalence of chronic illness on the financing and organization of home care are noted.

Chapter Three describes various features of the American health care system as they relate to some attributes of the nation, such as its size and demographic composition. Medicare

1

and Medicaid are then discussed, as are various criticisms of these programs.

In Chapter Four, we review some features of the acute care model of illness that dominates the American health care system. We analyze some important characteristics of the current criticisms of the health care system in terms of how it meets the problems of the disabled and the chronically ill. We then touch on some potential weaknesses in approaches to policy issues represented by the critics of the current system.

1

✳ ✳ ✳ ✳ ✳

Introduction:
New Perspectives
on the Implications
of Chronic Illness

We believe that new modes of thinking about chronic illness are needed that will bring effective medical care and nursing to the realities of lifelong illnesses. Existing perspectives on chronic illness are major barriers to these new ways of thinking. Professional perspectives must be altered before the American health care system can meet the requirements of a citizenry suffering disproportionately from chronic diseases. One reason the ill suffer is our current inability to cure or even mitigate some illnesses. Another reason, however, is that current organizational arrangements, whether public or private, are strikingly inadequate, hence unintentionally brutal. Lay perspectives on chronic illness and its treatment are mostly reflective of professional ones; the wider public too needs to understand the deeper implications of contemporary chronic illness.

Current debate about what is wrong with our health care system is, of course, vigorous and complex, covering a spectrum of issues: cost, technological assessment, equity, bioethics, and so on. Entering into this debate are perspectives that themselves are deeply—perhaps fatally—affected by modes of thinking and health organization that are far less pertinent to the management of chronic illnesses than acute ones. These perspectives, however varied they seem, rest on assumptions that ultimately lead to a dead end. Even those people who advocate increasing the funding of home care and expanding the availability of psychological and other kinds of counseling do not go far enough in their advocacy and their criticism of current health care arrangements. They too are trapped by the dominant image of acute illness and its concomitant physician-dominated care.

Much of the critical policy writing on chronic illness has been done by those who are involved in gerontological or rehabilitation services and policy writing: most nonclinical research that bears on the chronically ill has been directed toward understanding the problems of older Americans. While the elderly are subject to many of the same health problems as younger Americans, their experience is not representative of the entire spectrum of chronic illness. The elderly are of course more likely than the others to be widowed, be retired from paid employment, and have adult and even middle-aged children. As a group, they have greater savings than younger people and they can utilize Medicare, but they also are more likely to have multiple chronic illnesses and functional disabilities. Moreover, the researchers and practitioners who have written about the elderly ill have looked primarily at visibly deteriorating or dying people. They have thought less about those whose physical conditions are stable (even if death from the illness is inevitable, as in the case of some children with cystic fibrosis) or those who make quick and sometimes repeated comebacks to stability after acute periods of illness (as in arthritis and diabetes). An illness may pass through several phases—acute, comeback, stable, unstable, deteriorating, and dying. Models or perspectives derived from observations of and research on the elderly are likely to be somewhat biased and unrepresentative of all chronic illness experience. Criticisms of these perspectives are discussed further in Chapter Four.

The position argued in this book rests on a theoretical framework that we call a *trajectory* model, discussed at length in Chapter Five. The key points in our position are outlined below.

First, chronic illness, rather than infectious or parasitic illness, is now the prevalent form.

Second, these illnesses—presumably incurable—may appear at any age, some people being born with one or more of them, although most people experience them later in life.

Third, chronic illnesses are for life—the ill must therefore think in terms of managing a lifelong course of illness.

Fourth, anyone with a chronic illness is likely to experience, over a lifetime, two or more of the following phases of illness: acute, comeback, stable, unstable, deteriorating, and dying.

Fifth, the acute phase of an illness is usually managed— in a hospital, if the illness is severe—by physicians and other health workers, who attempt to stabilize the illness physiologically and promote the beginnings of a comeback from the acute state.

Sixth, the management of all phases of most chronic illness—except for the most acute and perhaps severely deteriorating phases—takes place at home. This management at home is carried out with the help of medical advice: it utilizes medical regimens, and it is abetted by visits to the physician's office or the clinic, or, more drastically, by occasional hospitalizations. Yet the day-in, day-out management must be done by the ill themselves, with the help, if necessary, of marital partners or other intimates, if available. Attempts to maintain a relatively stable state, as far as this is possible, make evident the centrality of stable phases in the work of managing chronic illness.

Seventh, a chronic illness and its management can and often do profoundly affect the lives and identities of the ill and their families—financially, emotionally, sexually, and, of course, in terms of running a household or raising children.

Eighth, as many people have argued, the needs of the ill and their families therefore encompass far more than the merely medical, even when an illness appears to be physiologically stable. The ill and their intimates can profit from counsel that goes far beyond what most physicians and nurses are trained to give.

Ninth, the current state of home care services is—as informed professionals and certainly many of the ill know—entirely inadequate. The primary reason is the acute care, medical perspective, dominant among health professionals and laypeople alike, which places health care facilities and their many resources at the center of health care. In this perspective, home care is seen only as secondary to this complex of technological-medical institutions.

Tenth, given the above considerations, a drastic rearrangement of institutions and funding of services is called for. The emphasis must be shifted much further toward home care.

Eleventh, the illness management done by the ill and their families at home is not simply a supplement to what the practitioners can do for them. It is central to a health care system that will effectively manage chronic illness. Care at home should be the center of the system and services should feed into and support the crucial work being done there.

Critics of the current health care system will recognize that our argument and its implicit trajectory model are suggesting some of the same correctives that can be found in the literature. Yet we claim that professional perspectives (and often gerontological ones) lead to somewhat less radical critiques than ours. Models that emphasize "patient/family responsibilities," matching professional services with "patients' needs," and even something as close to the trajectory model as a "client-based service model" do not encompass the fuller implications of what the prevalence of chronic illness means either for the health services or for the ill and their families themselves. As we argue more elaborately in Chapter Four, a professionalized and rather intellectualized, "top-down" perspective on health care is still dominant. Listening closely to the ill themselves leads to a more grass-roots approach that leaves ample room for—and recognizes the importance of—health professionals and legislative and other experts in the total division of labor.

2

✳ ✳ ✳ ✳ ✳

The Prevalence
and Complex Nature
of Chronic Illness

Though it is hardly as dramatic as the arrival of the atomic bomb and the threat of nuclear warfare, there is unquestionably something startling about the biological condition of a considerable and increasing portion of the earth's population: namely, the prevalence of the chronic rather than the acute illnesses. In this book, we argue that although some implications of that prevalence for health care are being increasingly recognized and are reshaping our health institutions and practices (note the impact of acquired immunodeficiency syndrome—AIDS—and Alzheimer's disease, for instance), neither the general public nor the health professionals recognize anything like the full implications of chronic illness for care, financing, insurance, the training of practitioners, or indeed for health facilities themselves. We are just beginning to pass into a period when chronic illness per se, rather than specific chronic diseases or categories of diseases, is referred to, thought about, and acted upon as a general reality rather than as a varied set of illness categories.

Defining Chronic Illness

It is surely because of their present incurability that these diseases are defined medically as chronic. Yet although some observers, including the famous Commission on Chronic Disease (Mayo, 1956), have recognized for at least three decades that they are the prevalent forms of illness, there is not even agreement on precisely what the term *chronic illness* means. Curtin and Lubkin have noted this lack of agreement in a concise and critical review of several well-known definitions (1986, pp. 5–6). For instance, they summarize Feldman's (1974) definition of chronic illnesses thus: "Ongoing medical conditions with spectrum of social, economic and behavioral complications that require meaningful and continuous personal and professional involvement." Curtin and Lubkin criticize this definition as more cognizant of the caretaker's role than the client's role. They summarize the views of Cluff (1981) this way: "A condition not cured by medical intervention requiring periodic monitoring and supportive care to reduce the degree of illness, maximize the person's functioning and responsibility for self-care." They remark that this view is somewhat medically oriented. The definition offered by Bauwens, Anderson, and Buergin (1983) is summarized thus: "Symptoms and signs caused by a disease within a variable period of time that runs a long course and from which recovery is only partial." Curtin and Lubkin comment that this view of chronic illness is disease-oriented. Curtin and Lubkin themselves are nurses and advocates of much-expanded home services to the chronically ill. They broaden the definition thus: "*Chronic illness* is the irreversible presence, accumulation, or latency of disease states or impairments that involve the total human environment for supportive care and self-care, maintenance of function, and prevention of further disability" (Curtin and Lubkin, 1986, p. 6). This definition captures the importance of the ill themselves and their families as well as that of the health services in the management of presently incurable, long-term illness that impinges on lives because it brings about—among other consequences—physical and mental disability.

Much of what has been written about the impact of chronic illness on activities, family life, and identity is also true of what is commonly referred to as physical or mental disability. The regimens for some chronic illnesses, like stroke and arthritis, imply the assistance of physical rehabilitation services. However, an accident to one's body is different from a disease, unless it also affects organs or bodily systems so as to bring about an illness. Of course, a severe accident, such as one that results in quadriplegia, will almost certainly also lead to one or more chronic conditions.

There is a similar definitional confusion about the terms *handicap* and *impairment*. As Schank (1986, p. 352) notes, "Rehabilitation definitions all speak to the problems of disability, and many relate to the handicapped or use words such as 'impairment' to indicate some decrease in function. Absence of clear differentiation among these terms causes confusion: which indicates decreased function without incapacitating the individual, and which refers to being incapacitated? There are times when the words are used interchangeably."

Even the term *physical limitation,* used in various surveys of chronic illness to measure the degree of disability among Americans, turns out on close scrutiny to mean different phenomena to different people, thus involving different criteria and therefore different objects of measurement. Ware (1986) has usefully summarized and cited much of the relevant literature. In studies and writings, the term *physical limitation* has variously referred to physical limitations, physical abilities, days in bed, mental anxiety and depression, psychological well-being, behavioral and emotional control, social visits with friends and relatives, telephone contacts, close friends, role functioning, current health, physical symptoms, and psychophysiological symptoms.

Perhaps the conclusion to be drawn about just how many people suffer one or more disabilities from a chronic illness is that the available statistics should be treated with some caution. Nevertheless, they give some idea of the widespread prevalence of chronicity in the American population.

Prevalence of Chronic Illness

In advanced, industrialized nations until the late 1930s, as in Third World countries today, the prevailing and often the most terrible afflictions were due to bacteria and parasites— the so-called acute diseases. A dramatic change took place when antibiotics and various improved immunological measures turned out to be highly effective against many of the infectious and parasitic diseases. While those diseases still reign in the less fortunate countries, most people in highly industrialized countries who are sick suffer from chronic illnesses. They include the cancers, arthritis, cardiovascular conditions, and a host of others that are currently incurable and sometimes scarcely controllable. Men and women have always suffered from these diseases, of course, but they were never before the most prevalent illnesses. They are now the equivalent of the plagues and scourges of yesteryear. Chronic illnesses are what bring people to the doctor's office, the clinic, and the hospital; they are what most people in developed nations die from. They are also, however, what people have to live with and manage at home on a day-to-day basis. As Brody, Poulshock, and Masciocchi wrote some years ago (1978, p. 556): "Chronic care is a major health problem of this generation. . . . Moreover, the rate of increase for funding long-term institutional care is more rapid in a health care system whose fiscal incentives are primarily responsive to acute care. . . . Indeed, much of the acute care delivered in short-term general hospitals is in response to acute episodes of chronic illnesses."

In the public mind, the illnesses associated with cancer, heart conditions, arthritis, and so on afflict people as they enter their fifties and later. In the most general sense, it is true that the elderly account for a disporportionate number of the illnesses.

Table 1. Percentage of the Population Limited in a Major Activity by Chronic Illness, by Age Group.

Age	Percentage Limited
All ages	9.4%
Under 18	3.6
18–44	5.7
45–64	17.8
65 +	22.7
65–69	30.1
70 +	18.9

Source: Adapted from Dawson and Adams, 1987, pp. 109–110.

Table 2. Percentage of the Population Limited in a Major
Activity by Chronic Illness, by Age Group and Level of Income.

Age	Percentage Limited			
	Under $10,000	$10–19,999	$29–34,999	$35,000 +
All ages	18.0%	12.0%	7.0%	5.2%
Under 18	5.6	4.3	3.0	2.9
18–44	10.9	7.4	4.9	3.7
45–64	45.7	24.6	14.4	8.9
65–69	45.6	33.7	21.9	20.8
70 +	24.0	16.4	13.1	15.3

Source: Adapted from Dawson and Adams, 1987, pp. 109–110.

As Tables 1 and 2 show, however, there is plenty of illness during the middle years, and the very young do not always escape disabling illnesses, including genetically derived heart defects and illnesses such as cystic fibrosis. The tables also suggest the considerable prevalence of chronic illnesses among the general population. While these illnesses tend to appear in the later years, they are nevertheless a threat for many people at any age. Note, however, that poor and less affluent Americans suffer more chronic illness in every age group.

Characteristics of Chronic Illness

Chronic illnesses share a number of prominent characteristics. They tend to be multiple diseases; they are long-term; they follow an uncertain course, often requiring large efforts at palliation; they are disproportionately intrusive upon the lives of the ill and their families; and they are expensive to treat and manage. Chronic illnesses also require a wide variety of ancillary services if they are to be properly cared for; they often imply conflicts of interpretation and authority among patients, family members, health workers, and funding agents; and they mainly require primary care (Gerson and Strauss, 1975, pp. 12–18; see also La Vor, 1979, pp. 26–28).

Multiple Chronic Illnesses. In 1971 it was estimated that 2.2 percent of Americans had multiple chronic conditions (U.S.

Department of Health, Education, and Welfare, 1971). Indeed, among the people whom we studied, they are quite frequent. Rice and La Plante (1986), comparing figures from 1969–1971 and 1979–1981, recently calculated that multiple conditions have increased significantly over the last decades. They conclude that "with declining mortality we appear to be seeing increasing morbidity, especially of disabling conditions that begin at the middle years and may extend into the future" (p. 21). Older people are more likely to have a higher rate of multiple diseases. As Butler and Newacheck (1981) note, there is also a higher incidence of chronic disease and disability among older women, especially those who are single.

Sometimes such chronic conditions are independent of each other, but of course sometimes they are closely linked. For a variety of reasons, long-term illnesses tend to multiply themselves, a single chronic condition often leading to multiple chronic conditions. First, many chronic illnesses are systemic or degenerative in effect, so that the long-term breakdown of one organ or physiological system leads to the involvement of others. Thus, for example, there are frequently connections among renal failure, certain cardiovascular involvements, and diabetes—the diabetes often leading to the other conditions. Second, the long-term disability or morbidity associated with chronic illness creates greater susceptibility to additional illnesses. Finally, the use of extremely powerful chemotherapeutic agents and radical surgical procedures as treatments for one chronic condition often causes additional iatrogenic disability.

Multiple conditions imply a multiplication of management problems, both at health care facilities and at home, as various treatment and management options for individual conditions are precluded by the additional disease-induced limitations. The multiplication of symptoms often curtails the abilities of the ill and their families to adjust to and compensate for limitations. Thus, a series of minor partial disabilities can interlock with one another to become, effectively, a near-total disability. This is exacerbated by the increasing psychological stress experienced by the sick person watching his or her body falling apart despite (or occasionally because of) the efforts of health workers. Often, the stress itself contributes to medical complications, as in syndromes involving hypertension. When a supportive network, whether of family or friends, fails, the ill are more likely to be institutionalized (Butler, 1977–1978). For instance, Butler and Newacheck (1981) report that widows and widowers are five times more likely to be institutionalized than those who are married; among the elderly, those divorced, separated, or never married have a rate of institutionalization that is even higher.

Long-Term Illness. The treatment of an acute disease usually takes days or weeks; rarely does it span months. Often, significant differences in a patient's condition can be achieved within hours or days of the start of medical care. The long-term character of chronic illness, by contrast, requires a form of health care organization suitable for repeated interaction over months and years between patients and health workers, and for the complex social relationships that grow up between them over the course of illness. The same is true—as we shall see graphically illustrated in our case materials—for the family's organization.

Uncertainty. Chronic illnesses tend to be uncertain in many ways. To begin with, the prognosis is often uncertain, and only the evolving course of the disease provides enough information to make possible a reasonable estimate of what is going to happen and when. Lupus is a striking example: the diagnosis is made an average of eight years after onset, and predicting the course of the illness and the effects of treatment is very difficult (Labrie, 1986). The same is true of many other chronic conditions. Such uncertainty can often cause considerable stress for patients (Locker, 1983; Wiener, 1975) and medical workers alike. At home, the inability to make long-range plans contributes an additional burden especially among young and middle-aged people, who have the bulk of their major life decisions still before them. In addition, the ill sometimes find themselves participating in the development of "frontier" medical technology when physicians use new drugs, devices, equipment, and surgical procedures in an attempt to bring the illness under control. The very existence of major research or experimental efforts contributes to additional uncertainty about the long-term course of an illness.

Furthermore, many illnesses are inherently episodic in nature; acute flare-ups are followed by apparent "remissions" or quiescent periods (Locker, 1983). Often the crises themselves are not predictable, and both the ill and the medical workers must be prepared for them at any time (Massie and Massie, 1973). The variety of uncertainties present in many illnesses forces the ill and their families to reorganize and restrict their lives in a continuing attempt to prepare for the unpredictable. Thus planning, both short- and long-term, is often extremely difficult. One of the most striking features of chronic illnesses is that they often require recurrent and unpredictable hospitalizations. A substantial proportion of people with chronic illnesses are likely to return to the hospital again and again whenever their illnesses become acute. The situation of the chronically ill can be seen as an oscillation between two poles: the home and the hospital (Strauss, Fagerhaugh, Suczek, and Wiener, 1985). Those who are extremely lucky need only to visit clinics or physicians' offices.

The phases of chronic illness (Vladeck, 1985) can usefully be classified with the following terms: acute, comeback, stable, unstable, deteriorating, dying (Corbin and Strauss, 1988). The *acute* phase includes crises or emergencies and their aftermath, as well as the active periods of an illness like arthritis. Acute phases are usually, but not always, managed within hospitals or other health facilities. Physiological *comeback*, or recovery, begins there, but comeback at home is both physiological and psychological. It is likely to require much time and work and to involve considerable interpersonal subtlety. *Stable* phases, as we shall see, seem simple; in fact, however, a great deal of work with regimens and the management of life's daily arrangements may be necessary just to stay stable. *Unstable* phases are periods when the patient's condition fluctuates continually without necessarily becoming acute. Living a normal life is then almost impossible. *Deterioration* of physical condition can proceed at varying rates. It affects the amount and kind of rearrangement necessary to maintain one's daily work and social life. The final phase, *dying,* scarcely needs to be mentioned at this point.

Intrusiveness. It must be emphasized that these chronic conditions are apt to be very intrusive on the lives of the ill and their families. Adjustment to the demands of regimens, and to the limits on activity imposed by symptoms or by the regimens themselves, requires a reorganization—often radical—of life-style, commitments, and activities. Because the illness is long-term in character, the sick person cannot drop out of normal activities temporarily. He or she must make major structural changes in how life is conducted. Sometimes these changes involve large costs to the ill and their associates.

Household routines, for instance, must often be rearranged to accommodate limitations on activity, the use of special equipment, the demands of the symptoms, or the scheduling of the regimen. This in turn affects the lives of other household members, requiring changes in how they manage their activities. These changes, combined with the frequent changes (for worse or better) in physical appearance, energy, and temperament that sick persons undergo, can greatly affect family relationships.

Cost. It is important to understand that even when extremely elaborate and expensive technologies are not normally used, the need for routine monitoring, the potential or actual crises, the use of drugs over long periods of time, and the extensive interaction with health facilities make caring for chronic illnesses expensive (Rice and Hodgson, 1981; Cluff, 1981). In addition, the complex and multiple nature of many chronic illnesses, as well as the need for a variety of ancillary health services, drives up substantially the direct costs of chronic illness care. Further, the opportunity costs of chronic illness are very high in comparison to infectious or parasitic illnesses; lost work alone can require sick Americans to become welfare recipients, and of course the restriction of activity often attendant on chronic illness means the sacrifice of recreational activities, even inexpensive ones. Furthermore, the long-term, repetitive, and complex character of chronic illness care naturally implies a greater

overhead and administrative costs for the ill, health organizations, and funding agencies alike. American families have been
forced by the extraordinary continuing expenses of some illnesses
to consume their savings and even to become welfare recipients
(Neifing, 1986).

Implications for the Ill, Their
Families, and Health Care Delivery

The social side effects of illness—whether derived from
financial issues or not—are at the very heart of what happens
at home, as the ill attempt both to manage their illnesses and
to stay on top of life itself. As our case materials amply illustrate,
these side effects lead inescapably to the conclusion that the ill
and their families require much more than medical counseling
and procedures (Lubkin, 1986). Their needs may be financial,
legal, or sexual; they frequently pertain to matters that are
marital or psychological or related to individual family members'
identities, as well as requiring assistance in physical matters such
as transportation or doing household chores. Chapter Three
discusses the general criticism of America's health care failings
in exactly this regard.

Health care personnel, social workers, rehabilitation specialists, and others prepare the acutely ill person to go home
from the hospital. Then they largely forget about him or her
until a medical or personal crisis brings the ill person back into
the health care or social service system once again. After the
acute and early rehabilitation phases of illness have passed, there
is little follow-up or follow-through by practitioners, except
perhaps in transplants and some rehabilitation programs, where
the need for a comprehensive and long-term approach to care
has generally been better understood.

Because of their acute care orientation, as well as their
work schedules, few nurses and probably fewer physicians are
equipped to provide multifaceted assistance. The medical literature is almost totally clinical in focus. The nursing literature
has begun to focus on the multiple needs of sick people at home
only in very recent years. Much of the writing about the chronic-

ally ill is still oriented to their clinical care. In one publication on chronic illness, the handbook opens with a pluralistic approach, but then each succeeding chapter is almost wholly clinically oriented. However, a book edited by Lubkin (1986) self-consciously downplays the clinical and focuses almost wholly on such important issues as mobility, funding, accessibility to agencies, sexual counseling, marital difficulties, and the like. In the next chapter, we will see how the current system for handling prevalent and complex chronic illnesses came to be.

3

✶ ✶ ✶ ✶ ✶

How the Health Care System Has Responded to Chronic Illness

Every country gets the health care system it deserves by virtue of the nature of the country—its demographic composition, forms of government, predominant types of economy, and so on. So it is inadvisable to attempt to understand, let alone explain, the character of the American health system by confronting it too directly. One cannot really understand the American health care scene if one approaches it without first putting it into a larger national context. For instance, nowadays it is common to refer to the nation's "health industry," noting that it has grown to be one of our largest industries. We may even believe that it is, or should be, directed largely by market forces—or argue, on the contrary, that health services cannot be conceived of as an industry because health is not simply a commodity and quality care cannot be measured in dollars. (In our discussion here, and throughout this book, we shall be focused on what is sometimes termed *the medical care system*. This discussion will omit the public health services, essential as these are, of course, to the nation's health.) If the latter view is true, why then do so many Americans speak of a health industry and why has the federal government recently acted so forcefully in terms of that economic imagery? Why do some people assert that America does not even have a health care "system," since health

18

services seem to present such a chaotic picture? Indeed, why is there such a diversity of views about what is currently wrong with the health care system and how it should be altered?

The American Health Care System

We shall take the precaution of pointing to a few structural and ideological features of the United States that affect both the unique shape of its health services and the different ways in which they are regarded (see also Anderson, 1985; Kaufman, 1987; Mechanic, 1986). That these features are crucial will immediately be clear, although to discuss the full details of their influence would deflect us from the purpose of this book. To begin with, the continental size of this country, the diversity of its many regions, and the large number of different ethnic traditions create a great diversity of perspectives and practices in health care, as in everything else. The size and diversity of the population and the affluence of the country permit a great number of vastly different facilities.

The American political system is a federal one, so health care is funded and regulated at every level of government: federal, state, county, and city. An unusually well developed commitment to voluntary action and voluntary organizations adds to the economic and political diversity of health facilities, and to the variety of groups such as self-help organizations (Cole, O'Conner, and Bennett, 1979; Gartner and Riessman, 1984; Mace and Babins, 1981) and fund-raising associations supportive of various medical specialties. The highly industrialized character of our economy also affects health services, especially in their use of sophisticated medical technology (equipment, drugs, medical supplies) produced and sold by a variety of profit-making companies (Roth and Ruzek, 1986; Schroeder and Showstack, 1979). In health care facilities, this technology is used with a high level of skill and knowledge by increasingly numerous technicians and medical and nursing specialists. The bulk of this technology, especially the most sophisticated and expensive, is used in hospitals (Strauss, Fagerhaugh, Suczek, and Wiener, 1985). These are at the center of the whole system of medical care.

Another major feature of this country is its socioeconomic stratification. Without getting into the lively debate on the exact character of that stratification, it is clear that a high proportion of our population enjoys relative economic security unless it is hit by catastrophic illness or the country suffers a severe depression. However, there is also a sizable proportion at any given time that has a very low income or that receives welfare support from our well-established, if much-criticized, welfare system. Historically, this characteristic socioeconomic division has furthered a two-tier system of health care, in which county hospitals serve the poorer population. Consequently, there has been a continuous struggle for a more equitable distribution of health care. This inequity of care undoubtedly still exists to a considerable degree (Davis and Rowland, 1983; Kasper, Walden, and Wilensky, 1978; Wilensky and Berk, 1982).

Yet another structural feature that affects the shape of our health services is America's mixed political economy, part free enterprise and part welfare state. This has assuredly contributed strongly to the unusual phenomenon of a highly industrialized and affluent country lacking state-financed and state-regulated national health insurance for its citizens. Rather, as a result of vigorous political maneuvering, the United States has evolved a flourishing health insurance industry that sells coverage to persons and groups. Side by side with this industry are publicly funded health services, like the Veterans Administration and those provided to some civil servants. Additionally, provision for the elderly and the poor is made through the government-funded programs of Medicare and Medicaid (Fein, 1981, 1986; Mechanic, 1986).

The American ideology of individualism also contributes to the general conviction that every American bears a large responsibility for his or her own health (self-care) as well as having the right to choose health services freely. Finally, there is the demographic composition of the United States. As everyone knows, the increasing numbers of people over the age of sixty-five ("the elderly," "young elderly," "old elderly," "over eighties," "over one hundred") are affecting the health care system directly and indirectly, through the changing composition of patients at health facilities (Estes and Lee, 1986; Vladeck and Firman, 1983) and through the pressure the elderly are increasingly able to exert on legislators regarding the distribution of health services.

What are the lineaments of the health care system—what health services are available to Americans, and how? The answer to that question depends in part on the position of whoever is characterizing the system. Our own perspective is shaped by our intention of indicating features of the health care system that affect and are affected by chronic illness. We can all agree, however, on the features of American health care arrangements named above: the number and diversity of health facilities, the public and private funding of facilities, much regulation by various levels of government, a diversity of technicians and specialists who contribute to the high quality of care, the use of sophisticated technology and supporting industries that produce this technology, the predominance of the hospital, a mixed system of private and public insurance, and a considerable socioeconomic inequity in accessibility to care and also to "quality" care.

Other features of the health care system that should be mentioned include the agencies that offer home care and the various rehabilitation services. (Both will be discussed later.) Two other visible and vital parts of our care system are the training programs and specialized schools for health care workers, and also the numerous, highly successful, and still evolving biomedical research institutions. A far less visible aspect of the care system consists of the countless caretakers of the chronically ill, principally their spouses, daughters, daughters-in-law, and parents (Brody, 1981; Coleman, Summers, and Leonard, 1982; Crossman, London, and Barry, 1981; Fengler and Goodrich, 1979). "Continuing research has shown that between two-thirds and three-quarters of the disabled elderly are cared for at home with few or no formal services" (Vladeck, 1985, p. 9).

At the fringes of the officially recognized health care system are a great many alternative care practitioners who are almost totally disregarded in policy discussions about America's health (Haldeman, 1980; Kaslof, 1978; Wolpe, 1985; Neuberger and Woods, 1986). It is to them that the ill turn, either initially or when they feel that standardized medicine has failed them. Among the alternative practitioners whom Americans can choose from are osteopaths, chiropractors, acupuncturists, and others who mainly treat psychological and mental problems. This list includes those, like the Chinese herbalists, who follow ethnically based practices. Many of these practitioners, who of course do not work at the usual health care facilities, have their own training programs and their own supportive supply companies. Like the domestic caretakers noted above, they are giving service—good, bad, or indifferent—to the chronically ill. Recognized or not by the medical profession or by legislative licensing, they are all but officially very much a part of our health care system.

Chronic Illness Shapes the Health Care System

The rapid increase of chronic illness prevalence since the 1950s, largely as a result of the use of antibiotics, has transformed our care system. That transformation is most obvious in the striking evolution of new medical, nursing, and biotechnical specialties. The explosion of knowledge, its base in supporting research, and its institutional base have resulted in numerous subspecialties, such as intensive care units (ICUs) and intensive care nurseries (Wiener, Fagerhaugh, Suczek, and Strauss, 1979; Guillemin and Holstrom, 1986). As an organizational form, the ICU is about thirty years old. It has not only become a basic part of the acute care hospital but has proliferated with subspecialties of its own, such as cardiac, neurological, and pediatric intensive care. There has been a similar evolution in the more complex clinics, even in those devoted to particular illnesses.

An equally striking response to the prevalence of chronic illness, and one that profoundly affects the kind, amount, and quality of care received by the elderly chronically ill, is the development of Medicare and Medicaid, the two central government-funded programs in our care system (Fein, 1986, pp. 52–124, 193–215). Brody (1987) has offered a useful three-stage description that emphasizes the historical evolution of these two programs. He argues that "the keystone of public policy for the aged during the last fifty years has been the avoidance of economic catastrophe for the aging family" (p. 131). The first perception of catastrophe—"the need for basic subsistence" (p. 131)—occurred during the Great Depression of the 1930s, and led to the setting up of Social Security. The second perception of catastrophe was that older people had "a lack of resources with which to purchase acute medical care" (p. 132). Publicly supported medical services had been developed in association with a reform movement during the progressive movement early in this century, but Medicare was not enacted until 1965. By then, 10 percent of the population was elderly. One elderly person out of six "was hospitalized at least once a year, with length of stay at least twice as long as for people under sixty-five years of age. . . . The catastrophe was defined primarily in terms of the cost of hospital care: and Medicare was the political solution" (p. 133). (Primarily, of course, people were hospitalized for acute phases of chronic illness or because their chronic conditions were considered to need surgery.) The third perception of catastrophe occurred still later: "Unnoticed at first, the third category, long-term care, was in its formative stages" (p. 134).

Brody shows the delayed societal response to disabilities in the elderly by comparing the 1910 Flexner report on medical education, which was thirty years in advance of the development of a firm scientific base for modern medicine, with the development of the recognition of long-term illness: "So did the 1956 Commission on Chronic Disease anticipate the beginning of the need for a societal response to disability by a similar time period. . . . Perception of catastrophe in economic terms is the sine qua non [in the United States] for policy change" (p. 134). In short, for the past fifteen years the nation has been struggling for a coherent policy to meet the economic needs of the chronically ill elderly. Brody realizes full well that this perception of a third economic catastrophe is still not widely enough recognized to give a strong political push to the attempts at reforming what the critics who share a long-term care perspective generally agree is wrong with the health care system. Medicare, as Vladeck (1983, p. 2) notes, "whatever the initial intent or language, was not in the long-term care business." From 1966 to 1968, Medicare supported "a substantial volume" of long-term care services, but the government later pulled back from that policy.

More recently, there has been legislative and executive alarm over the increasing numbers of the elderly and what that increase might portend if the government seriously got into the funding of long-term care. Estes and Lee (1986) sum up the current situation concisely, comparing what Medicare does with what it does not do: "Although Medicare has been the most important source of payments for hospitals and physicians caring for the elderly since 1965, it is limited in scope of benefits and reimbursement policies required to meet the needs of the chronically ill and disabled elderly. The cost of care, that is, the full range of services addressing the health, personal, and social needs, is borne by both the private (the elderly themselves and their families) and the public sectors" (p. 344).

Yet, as Vladeck (1985, p. 13) notes, "Medicare is implicated in the long-term care system to a far greater extent than is generally recognized." For instance, Medicare pays for a great many services to the chronically ill that have not been "systematically identified as [services]." Among these are the fees paid to physicians who visit nursing homes and home care patients. Vladeck notes that a significant though unknown number of Medicare hospital admissions are from nursing homes and are often linked with inadequate or insufficient care there; he also points out that 3–7 percent of all Medicare patients with acute care status are awaiting nursing home placement.

Before the mid 1970s, long-term care for the elderly was essentially equivalent to nursing home care. In 1975–76, "it became clear that nursing homes were receiving 90 percent of all, and 98 percent of public, long-term dollars" (Vladeck, 1983, p. 1). It also became evident that Medicaid was carrying most of this financial burden. Medicaid had been conceived of as an adjunct to welfare programs covering health insurance for recipients of Aid to Families with Dependent Children. By the mid 1970s, it had become clear that "Medicaid was buying services for the frail elderly'' (Vladeck, 1983, p. 2). These people had never before been supported by a governmental agency.

Medicaid is mostly funded by the states. The financial crisis in recent years has brought about significant cutbacks in Medicaid. However, as might be expected, the funding now varies considerably from state to state (Estes and Lee, 1986, p. 344), as do the services covered (Neifing, 1986). Contributing to the cutbacks has been the Reagan administration's strategy of pulling back from Medicaid. Nevertheless, the Medicaid program continues to be the funding of last resort for catastrophic and long-term care insurance beneficiaries who are elderly. Vladeck (1985) sums it up in this way: ''Two essential points need to be made. First is the near-total interdependence of Medicare and Medicaid policies as they involve long-term care clients; when Medicare sneezes, Medicaid catches pneumonia. Second is the bizarre character of the Medicaid eligibility process for most long-term care clients. To oversimplify only slightly, Medicaid coverage of long-term care is provided largely to formerly middle-class people who have been totally impoverished by medical and related expenses, and is much more readily available to people already in nursing homes than equally poor and disabled people not in them. . . . Medicaid is quite literally the payer of last resort'' (pp. 15–16). It is for this reason that some writers have referred to ''the process of pauperization'' (Gerson and Strauss, 1975) and others to ''the cycle of poverty'' or similar terms when considering the plight of working-class or middle-class people who are faced with a long-term catastrophic illness. It is important to note that the ill who are under sixty-five years of age do not have Medicare support.

A large percentage of the American population is covered by private or public insurance plans. These plans, however, are notably deficient in a number of ways in their coverage of catastrophic physical or mental illness. Furthermore, the poorest Americans (including many black Americans and certain other minorities) suffer most from disabling chronic illness and are the least well insured (Davis and Rowland, 1983). Over 25 million people at any time, and as many as 35 million at some period during the year, may be uninsured by private insurance plans or public programs (Kasper, Walden, and Wilensky, 1978; Wilensky and Berk, 1982). "For many of the uninsured, community health centers and migrant health centers have helped to fill the gap in access created by the lack of insurance. These are especially important for those ineligible for Medicaid" (Davis and Rowland, 1983, p. 169). These programs have also suffered major cutbacks under the current federal administration. Even programs like the Social Services Block Grant and Older Americans Act, which support nonprofit voluntary agencies and "are a vital part of the long-term-care picture . . . garner considerably less public resources than the strictly medically defined long-term-care" (Estes and Lee, 1986, p. 344).

Recent lobbying and congressional response are leading to legislative action for catastrophic insurance coverage. This is directed mainly at the desirable goal of insurance for catastrophic acute illness and nursing home care. As long-term care proponents well understand, however, the aim of this particular legislation is only a first step toward much more extensive support for long-term care services.

The above quotations make quite clear what the advocates of long-term care (mostly focused on the problems of the elderly) think are the shortcomings of our particular system of health care. Before discussing their more specific criticisms, we will note a recent development that is especially pertinent to the chronically ill. This is what some observers have termed the "home care boom" (Neifing, 1986, p. 307; Vladeck, 1985). According to the National Home Care Association, there has been a 241 percent increase in home health agencies (Dunphy, 1984). Vladeck (1985) has noted that as the supply of nursing homes shrank after the nursing home scandals of the middle seventies, in-home services grew enormously. In 1980 and 1981, Medicare home health benefits were increased, and Medicaid benefits were "encouraged in 1981 legislation" (Vladeck, 1985, p. 6). Since then, "home health care has been the fastest-growing category of Medicare expenditures, with a compound annual growth rate in excess of 20 percent" (Vladeck, 1985, p. 6; U.S. General Accounting Office, 1982). Contributing to this increased concern with and development of health care services are the earlier discharges of patients from hospitals because of cost containment strategies. Extended care facilities and families have had to step in to handle these earlier discharges. Because of the added burden they place on family caretaking, some observers have been critical of the new governmental regulations and hospital responses. A skeptical observer can view the buildup of home care agencies as "poorly organized" and the result of "a desperate attempt to meet the needs of clients quickly and an opportunity to make money" (Neifing, 1986, p. 306).

The American health care system reflects several unique characteristics of this nation. As well, it has been shaped in recent years by the shift in prevalence from acute to chronic illnesses. It is important for us to understand that the long-term care aspects of our health care system—and the central funding programs of Medicare and Medicaid—suffer from a number of shortcomings in their provision for the chronically ill. In the next chapter, we will discuss specific problems of the prevailing acute care approach to illness in greater detail and the need for reform in the health care system.

4

∗ ∗ ∗ ∗ ∗

Why Major Reform
Is Needed

The predominantly clinical or acute care approach to chronic illness seems to be only partly relevant to the many nonclinical aspects of chronic illness, and to the cluster of problems that characteristically confront the chronically ill. The inability of the ill to surmount those problems and to manage the nonclinical aspects of their lives unquestionably contributes to their specifically medical difficulties. In this chapter, we consider the prevailing acute care approach to illness—including chronic illness—and various criticisms directed against this approach. We also contrast the ways that health professionals and laypeople perceive the issues of chronic illness.

Weaknesses of the Acute
Care Approach to Chronic Illness

Along with the gradual recognition by perceptive observers and researchers of the complex accompaniments of long-term illnesses, there has evolved a thoughtful criticism of the acute care approach to currently incurable illnesses (Brody, Poulshock, and Masciocchi, 1978; Conrad, 1987; Feldman, 1974; La Porte and Rubin, 1979). The tenor of criticism is exemplified by statements such as that of Leighton Cluff (1981), a physician and former executive vice-president of the Robert Wood Johnson

28

Foundation. Cluff points out the efficacy of the clinical approach to illness, then faults it for what it frequently fails to do: ''Medical knowledge and skill, diagnosis and treatment of disease, mortality and morbidity, pathophysiology and other similar concerns frequently dominate the interests and efforts of doctors. These concerns are important to the management of disease and contribute to functional improvement of patients. Too seldom, however, do physicians attend to the patient's ability to cope, level of discomfort, patterns of living, occupational ability or productivity, emotional status, or other functional activities'' (p. 306).

It is understandable that an acute care approach should predominate in hospitals, but why should it also characterize the care of patients at clinics and in physicians' offices? Some 52 percent of those who seek help in these places suffer from chronic illness (Rice and Hodgson, 1981). The answer perhaps lies in part in the overwhelming clinical emphasis of medical school faculties and, though to a rapidly lessening extent, in schools of nursing. A number of factors contribute to this clinical emphasis in the training of young physicians (Becker, Geer, Hughes, and Strauss, 1964). To be accepted into a medical school, students must have undergone an undergraduate education consisting mostly of courses in science. This concentrated premed curriculum will culminate—in their eyes—in the ''real thing'' when they finally engage in clinical work at a teaching hospital (Becker, Geer, Hughes, and Strauss, 1964). At medical school, their teachers are skilled and sometimes famous medical scientists and clinicians. The curriculum emphasizes the rigorous scientific basis (''hard science'') of good medical practice, and students are trained primarily in hospitals (Becker, Geer, Hughes, and Strauss, 1964). The school itself is located in a teaching hospital, most frequently devoted to the most acute kinds or phases of chronic illnesses. Students almost everywhere rank the prestige of the more socially and psychologically oriented specialties, such as psychiatry, family medicine, and rehabilitation medicine (Anderson, 1978), below that of the more rigorously clinical specialties. In recent years more attention has been paid to the social and psychological aspects of patient care, yet the teaching of these is likely to be squeezed out or minimized, if only because the specialties compete so ferociously for students and the medical curriculum requires so much concentrated study. During the even more intensive years of internship and residency, the postgraduate students are similarly wrapped up in clinical work and learning (Bucher and Stelling, 1977; Mizrahi, 1987).

Yet the clinical training of physicians cannot be the only reason that the medical-clinical perspective is so dominant at health care facilities. If medical leaders thought it was, they would do what the leaders of the nursing profession have done: emphasize the social and psychological aspects of care, even in the hospital setting, where the physicians control or influence so much of the operative policy. Perhaps, as some observers have suggested (Roth and Ruzek, 1986; Strauss, Fagerhaugh, Suczek, and Wiener, 1985; Wiener, Fagerhaugh, Suczek, and Strauss, 1979), the very success of modern medicine in combating disease and vanquishing particular diseases, abetted by the effectiveness of an explosively evolving technology, has persuaded both physicians and laypeople that what is needed is more medical science, more high-quality medicine, and further improved technology (Strauss, Fagerhaugh, Suczek, and Wiener, 1985; Wiener, Fagerhaugh, Suczek, and Strauss, 1979). With these, even more disease will be conquered (Thomas, 1974).

Indeed, it is difficult to talk about medical treatments without using military terminology, as several critics have pointed out (Schwartz, 1987; Childress, 1987; Vaisrub, 1977; Sontag, 1979; Warren, 1987). Childress (1987, pp. 486–487), a bioethicist, makes a strong case for the physicians' use of a "metaphor of warfare." In perhaps too extreme a statement but certainly with considerable truth, he sketches out the metaphor: "The physician as the captain leads the battle against disease, orders a battery of tests, develops a plan of attack, calls on the armamentarium or arsenal of medicine, directs allied health personnel, treats aggressively and expects compliance. Good patients are those who fight vigorously and refuse to give up. Victory is sought and defeat is feared. Sometimes there is even hope for a "magic bullet" or a "silver bullet." Only professionals who stand on the firing line or in the trenches can really appreciate the moral problems of medicine. As medicine wages war against germs that invade the body and threaten its defenses, so the society itself may also declare war on cancer under the leadership of its chief medical officer—the Surgeon General. Articles and books may even herald the 'Medical-Industrial Complex: Our National Defense.'

Although the acute care approach to illness has had many victories, it also has some crucially important negative consequences that militate against the more effective management of chronic illness—and certainly against a great success in improving the quality of life of the chronically ill. For example, the clinical approach leads directly to a faith in high-technology medicine, with its emphasis on intensive care carried out primarily in hospitals and secondarily in clinics. Hence, as noted earlier, the acute care hospital is the centerpiece of the contemporary health enterprise (Scott, 1972). Funding, whether federal or through insurance, goes primarily to support acute care facilities and medical practice. Only secondarily does funding go to support home care services. Critics like Childress (1987) suggest that the acute care perspective, expressed in military metaphor, leads physicians to assign "priority to *critical* care over prevention and chronic care. It tends to view health in negative rather than positive terms, as the absence of disease rather than a positive state of affairs, and concentrates on critical interventions to cure disease. . . . It tends to neglect care when cure is impossible" (p. 486). Or it saves people without concern for the quality of their lives once they are sent home.

The acute care perspective also emphasizes technology and downplays less technological modes of care. This is true despite the great difficulty of assessing the usefulness of particular types of technology, the considerable cost of some technologies, the probable overuse of some for particular patients, and the inevitable stopgap quality or "half-way technology" (Thomas, 1974, p. 16) of many. Even the funding available for medical research is skewed in the direction of "killer" illnesses; little attention is paid to less alarming but exceedingly important and widespread conditions like arthritis and disabilities derived from back trouble.

The mounting criticism of purely clinical medicine calls for ''an expansion in services geared to supportive maintenance, patient management, and new kinds of preventive care'' (Schwartz, 1987, pp. 485–486). Supportive services ''may contribute more to monitoring [patients'] functioning ability, while at the same time reducing the need for costly forms of care and assisting patients to remain or become economically independent and productive'' (Cluff, 1981, pp. 300–301).

These are criticisms to which we subscribe (Strauss and Glaser, 1975; Strauss, Fagerhaugh, Suczek, and Wiener, 1985; Corbin and Strauss, 1988). In fact, we believe, as do many other researchers, that even in hospitals there should be much more focus on the social and psychological aspects of care of the chronically ill, not only to facilitate their coming to terms with their illness but also to help them learn to live with it day by day, integrating the illness into their lives. Nurses and medical social workers have been moving steadily toward that position, while developing so-called clinical ''soft technologies'' to supplement the more obviously ''hard'' technologies. Yet even these professionals do not generally understand that, because their patients usually have histories of chronic illness, they are knowledgeable about their own illness management. This inevitably leads to tensions and conflicts between the hospital staffs and the patients. The latter then tend to be regarded as uncooperative or difficult. Meanwhile, many patients who have been hospitalized repeatedly believe that they can distinguish a competent nurse or technician from an incompetent one. Therefore, they may level specific accusations of incompetence or negligence against a staff member, based on what they believe are good experiential grounds (Fagerhaugh and Strauss, 1977). Nor do hospital personnel generally understand that these chronically ill patients do a great deal of illness management work in the hospital itself (they have, of course, been accustomed to doing this at home). This work includes monitoring staff members for their competence in giving safe care (Strauss, Fagerhaugh, Suczek, and Wiener, 1985; Fagerhaugh, Strauss, Suczek, and Wiener, 1987).

If this is so for the hospital situation, consider the consequences of applying the dominant acute care approach to patients after their return home. Although patients are given a regimen and advised to adhere to it, it is anticipated that some will only partly follow these regimens. Indeed, there is a sizable research and rhetorical literature about "recalcitrance"—the professionals' term for the apparently irrational or perverse actions of patients concerning their regimens (Sackett and Snow, 1979). "When this problem was first discovered, many practitioners responded with 'awestruck disbelief'" (Svarstad, 1976, p. 439). Despite the probably widespread views of physicians about this matter, researchers have demonstrated that the grounds on which patients judge their regimens are quite rational; patients weigh their personal concerns, the contingencies of their lives, and the perceived seriousness of the illness or symptoms against the time and effort the regimens require and the side effects they cause (Conrad, 1985; Becker and Maiman, 1975; Corbin and Strauss, 1985). Further, patients sometimes do not understand the regimens; staffs at the health facilities do not always explain them clearly, either because they do not realize that their explanations are unclear or because they are concentrating on problems of higher (usually clinical) priority (Levy, 1979). It is possible that patients' dissatisfaction with the physician who has counseled the regimen also affects their strict adherence to it (Svarstad, 1976).

Among nurses, there is an increasing emphasis on the necessity for teaching patients before their discharge from the hospital, and teaching the kin, too, if feasible. Yet the very organization of many hospital wards, especially in the intensive care units, militates against giving much priority to teaching efforts. A recent survey of practices within intensive care nurseries, combined with a careful ethnographic study of one intensive care nursery (Guillemin and Holstrom, 1986), portrays vividly the staff's dedication to the work of saving the lives of infants and their great skill in doing so. This research also shows how little effort generally is made to communicate more than superficially with the parents or to attend to their psychological problems—and how little training the staff members usually have in these matters (see also Wiener, Fagerhaugh, Suczek, and

Strauss, 1979). (Of course, some intensive care nurseries do have trained nursing care specialists who are keenly aware of such problems.) Consequently, we wonder what happens when these infants are returned to their parents, who must live with and manage whatever chronic illnesses may develop despite the heroic efforts of the intensive care staff. If this is characteristic of what occurs in hospitals, consider what then happens after a hospitalized patient returns home, given both the clinical orientation at the clinics and physicians' offices and the shape of the American health care system.

We have already noted (Chapter Three) that home care is an undernourished child of that system. This is understandable, given that the acute care perspective so profoundly colors the thinking of the physicians who are the dominant health care professionals (Freidson, 1970a), as well as that of other health professionals who work more or less under their aegis (Scott, 1972). Consequently, critics can point to what seems to be a clear mismatch between the organization of health care and the requirements of managing chronic illness (Schwartz, 1987; Vladeck, 1983). Despite such criticism, the continued strength of the acute care perspective should not be underestimated. It is more or less shared by the legislators and executives of the federal and state governments as well as by other lay citizens. Furthermore, Freidson (1986), who has been carefully following the evolution of the medical profession, suggests there will be further evolution of new or renovated forms of organized practice (health maintenance organizations, ambulatory surgical centers, and so on); as "is the case for hospitals and medical schools, representation in such associations is institutional in character, embodied in the directors, deans, or chief executive officers responsible for the institution as a whole" (p. 76). He argues that the orientation of these personnel is principally toward protecting their institution and its interests, with much consequent attention to the political and economic climate in which it operates, and with rather less concern with the everyday problems of giving patient care. Whether or not his prediction is correct—whether the officials or the physicians have the most influence—these facilities at the heart of the health care system (public health excepted) represent a very strong barrier to any radical shift of perspective on health care.

Criticisms and Suggestions

For many years, the nation's current health care arrangements have been subject to a barrage of criticism as experts and laypeople alike find fault with one or another feature of them. Indeed, with increasing acerbity and increasing numbers of players, a complex and passionately argued debate has been raging in the health care arena. It concerns the proper ways in which the health system should be organized and health care delivered. The current turmoil consequent on high medical costs and the increasingly severe regulation of hospitals and health practitioners have added to the complexity and passion of the debate. Issues of cost, quality care, bureaucratic constraints, accessibility to care, patient consent, the right to die, technological advances, and alarming technological by-products—all are now highly visible items in the news media. Moreover, it is probable that the debate will continue with unabated intensity for many years, exhibiting a further and sometimes bewildering array of panaceas, plans, programs, models, and suggestions.

The views of critics who assess the health system from the standpoint of its performance in long-term care, including their criticisms of the prevailing acute care approach, are especially pertinent to our own. We will discuss a few of their views and suggestions for improving long-term care. While there are differences of emphasis, there seems to be a consensus that the current arrangements fall far short of what is needed. Five major points on which there is relative agreement are summarized below.

First, long-term care involves far more than is offered in acute care facilities. Second, clinical care should be supplemented by services that will meet the rehabilitative, psychological, economic, social, and other needs of the ill. Third, there should be a shift in funding patterns so that these other services can be greatly expanded. Fourth, funding for the poor requires special attention, for they bear the burden of the health care system's failings; their care is less accessible and of lower quality, although the poor are more disabled and sicker than the rest of our population. Fifth, funding arrangements to cover potential economic catastrophe for all ill or disabled Americans are imperative.

There is general agreement, too, on the list of services that would make long-term care comprehensive, continuous, flexible, responsive to what the ill and disabled require, and respectful of them and their families. As Vladeck (1983, p. 7) remarks, these requirements "are hardly radical or unfamiliar to health care professionals," at least to those especially concerned with long-term care.

On the question of how to attain these goals there is somewhat less agreement. As might be anticipated, the diversity of suggestions for changing or supplementing the present system is affected by the different perspectives associated with professional positions and experiences. We will present a few of the suggestions made by people who have been much concerned with improving long-term care.

One suggestion for reform emphasizes the necessity to raise public awareness about the long-term care issue. This emphasis is largely a political one. It has been well stated by Brody, who argues that to get maximum changes in the desired direction now, "perception of catastrophe in economic terms is the *sine qua non* for policy change" (1987, p. 135). This implies that continuity of care needs to be stated "in specific terms which then can be costed out" (p. 135). Otherwise, we cannot effectively counter the argument of legislators and others who are frightened of the bottomless pit of potential expenditures and anticipate unending demands by the aged ill and disabled. These fears are fed by memories of the haste with which legislators responded to the lobbying of kidney dialysis proponents for carte blanche aid to kidney patients. Politicians must be convinced of what research has already clearly demonstrated: the families of the ill will not abdicate their responsibilities once adequate government funding is available.

Some critics believe that Americans more or less agree on what is wrong with the health care system but disagree on what should be changed. Therefore, reform efforts are mired.

"It may be that the current policy stalemate arises at root from value conflicts about the appropriate roles of government, families, and individual responsibility so profound that only creative and aggressive policy leadership, of a kind now nowhere to be found, can end it" (Vladeck, 1984, p. 2). Meltzer, Farrow, and Richman (1981, p. 6) make a similar point when they assert that "the most important policy problem is a lack of consensus about the nature and extent of public responsibility for meeting long-term-care needs. This results in an inability to articulate a single set of goals and directions for future policy development."

A more systematic and extended statement, based on careful research, is offered by Budrys (1986), who assesses the situation in this way: "The persistent perception of a health crisis stems from society's lack of confidence in the social control arrangements governing the activities of the health sector in recent years; what is worse the public is confused about who should be entrusted with the responsibility for planning the nation's health" (1986, p. 113). Budrys points to three different systems of control and responsibility. The first is the administrative approach; the second is the professional approach; and the third is the market approach. Each has strengths and weaknesses. In consequence, a typical cycle occurs. Budrys's description of it is this:

> The analogy that comes to mind to illustrate what has been happening in the health sector over the past few decades is that it has fallen into a deep circular rut from which we are now having difficulty extricating it. The circularity of this rut is caused by the following pattern: as each new health sector problem is identified, a mechanism (that is, an agency, incentive program, or such) is created to address it; a sizable number of people become involved in the operations of the mechanisms; after a short period of time some faction of observers begins pointing out its shortcomings and proposing alternatives; however, those involved in the operations of that mechanism have a stake in de-

fending it and do so; the rhetoric escalates; those
involved in the mechanism's operations eventually
start to become demoralized and move into other
parts of the health sector; the mechanism begins
to wither away from lack of support; meanwhile,
the problems that came to light while the mechanism in question was operative are thought to be
even more pressing; and a new mechanism is in-
troduced based on the presumed urgency of the
need for it, which brings another wave of participants whose interest in the operations of the newest
mechanism become quickly vested. And the circular
rut begins anew! The rut continues to grow deeper,
of course, with the increased weight of each new
wave of participants. Finding a way out of this rut,
obviously, does not become any easier with delay
[pp. 132–133].

Her solution is to blow the whistle on the debate—a vain solution, we believe—buckle down to rational consideration of the
inevitable strengths and weaknesses of each control system, "and
develop a higher level of [political] consensus regarding the
strengths and weaknesses of each before opting for changes in
current health care delivery arrangements" (1986, p. 133).

    A second suggestion for reform focuses on the inadequa-
cies of current funding mechanisms and how they might be rectified to give greater financial support to those who need long-
term care. When the focus is on the elderly ill and disabled or
the poor elderly, then the suggestions may refer to altering
Medicare or Medicaid. The tenor of such suggestions is con-
veyed by Davis and Rowland (1983, p. 525): "Medicaid coverage should be expanded to provide basic insurance coverage for
all low-income individuals . . . implementation of coverage for
the medically needy would be another step toward reducing
disparities between the South and the rest of the country."
Private insurance plans also ought to be modified, for example,

to compensate for the current link between unemployment and lack of health insurance coverage. Another suggestion is to experiment ''with capitation payments to individual primary care centers, networks of centers, hospitals, or other major primary care providers for providing ambulatory and in-patient services to Medicaid beneficiaries'' (Davis and Rowland, 1983, p. 525; see also Winn and McCaffree, 1979). The feasibility of public payments to families for their care giving is also being talked about and research on the matter is under way (Fengler and Goodrich, 1979; Arling and McAuley, 1983).

When the poor or particular deprived minorities are in focus, whether they are elderly or not, a third theme colors the policy suggestions. This pertains to equity, to fairness in access to quality health care. Equity has long been a primary agenda of those who represent the poor and minorities (Wiener, Fagerhaugh, Suczek, and Strauss, 1979; Davis and Rowland, 1983; Fein, 1986).

Other reform suggestions are more specific, centered on particular features of prevailing health care arrangements. For example, to get adequate and appropriate services, the ill have to find their way through a veritable ''agency maze,'' with its accompanying fragmentation, lack of communication between agencies and care givers, high costs for services, and agency politics (Friedemann, 1986; Harding, Heller, and Kesler, 1979; Waitzkin, 1983; Wheeler-Lachowycz, 1983; Feder, 1983). It is argued that this situation needs to be rectified by various organizational strategies. Or the rehabilitation services are believed to be inadequate in one or another regard, and this situation should be corrected (Schank, 1986; Becker and Kaufman, 1987; Verville, 1979; Fowler, 1982; Rothberg, 1981; Fordyce, 1976; Kaufman and Becker, 1986; Roth, 1984). Or the rehabilitation practitioners are viewed as typically not focused on chronic illnesses; they should be more aware of them and chronically ill patients should be referred to rehabilitation services by the physicians (Schank, 1986). Or the linkage between the hospital and the home health agencies is judged to be very poor and should be greatly strengthened (Strauss, Fagerhaugh, Suczek, and Wiener, 1985; Vladeck, 1984, p. 11; Jillings, 1987).

Or it is suggested that the connection between the formal services and the informal (family) ones needs to be carefully thought
through and worked out (Brody, 1981; Vladeck, 1983, p. 18).
Or nurses and others who visit the homes of the ill should pay
more attention to the social and psychological needs of the clients
and their caretakers; and, more generally, they should carefully
attempt to match services to the clients' needs (Hooyman,
Gonyea, and Montgomery, 1985) and to the care givers' needs
as well (Crossman, London, and Barry, 1981; Coleman, Summers, and Leonard, 1982).

In stating these typical positions and suggestions so baldly,
we do not mean to denigrate them. In fact, each certainly deserves careful consideration, and of course some are getting that
consideration rather widely.

Professional and Lay Approaches to Illness

The writings of the reform advocates cited above and
others like them have a common feature, despite differences in
their specific suggestions for improving long-term care. This
feature is their highly professionalized view of what is wrong
with organized health care arrangements. This should occasion
no surprise, since the authors all have had professional training, positions, and experience (Freidson, 1970a, 1970b, 1986;
Hughes, 1971). This does not mean they are insensitive to or
disrespectful of the viewpoints or wishes of the ill and their
families. Yet a professional perspective deeply colors the language even of those who advocate the most cooperative relationships with the ill. Often the ill are referred to as patients
or clients, which, from a professional's standpoint, of course,
they are. Therefore, we are offered suggestions for what amounts
to a patient centered professional model (Cluff, 1981, p. 2), a
"patient centered" model (Lubkin, 1986, p. 121), a "client
based perspective" (Vladeck, 1984, p. 1), and a "goal oriented
approach" to real-life functioning, rather than a predominantly
clinical approach. Programs are assessed for their matching of
services with "needs" of the ill (Vladeck, 1984, p. 2), and in
terms of a cause-effect model of the degree to which they are

effective, efficient, cost effective, and so on (Budrys, 1986, pp. 51–71; Fein, 1981).

This kind of terminology reflects an underlying specialist stance. It is markedly different from the attitude that can be sensed in the words and actions of some self-help groups (Maines, 1984), and the more militant disabled groups (Zola, 1981, 1982), as well as in writings derived from the concerns of the women's movement (Coleman, Summers, and Leonard, 1982; Lewin and Olesen, 1985). The perspectives of these groups surely are not those of health or rehabilitation professionals or professional gerontologists, nor of political scientists, social workers, or government administrators. Professionals and the lay disabled and ill are, of course, often able to act cooperatively in the political arena, yet their fundamental views are far from identical. We believe that the professionals' approach makes them insufficiently sensitive to some of the subtler issues involved in staying afloat when burdened with a severe chronic illness (Massie and Massie, 1973). This, of course, has some negative consequences for practitioners and policy approaches to the problems of the chronically ill (see Chapters Ten and Eleven).

Practitioner training is highly technical, with therapies and procedures that have been carefully assessed and at least partly related to professional philosophies of treatment (Becker, Geer, Hughes, and Strauss, 1964). Later experiences in the field, as practitioner, teacher, or researcher, build on a great deal of technical knowledge and skill. Further, a health professional almost always works in an organizational context. He or she inevitably must take elements of that context into account, whether they are agency requirements, intraagency and interagency relationships, legislative mandates and constraints, colleague relationships, or interdisciplinary working relationships (Scott, 1972).

A somewhat intellectualized approach to illness and its accompanying social and psychological patterns is contributed to both by this organizational context and by professional training and experience (Strauss, Fagerhaugh, Suczek, and Wiener, 1985; Guillemin and Holstrom, 1986). (We are not saying this is bad—only different.) This can be seen in nurses, physicians, and social workers even when someone in their own family becomes chronically ill; one cannot expect them to tear their professionalized approaches from their brains, nor would it make any sense if they did. The professionalized approach, however, is at some variance with the approaches of laypeople, except those who themselves have become considerably professionalized. Their worlds are not the professional's world, and vice versa. The ill and their families are concerned with managing the vagaries of illness, and with living with it and whatever regimens and limitations it entails. They are also concerned with managing living day to day with whatever resources they have and whatever arrangements can be set up and maintained.

An essentially top-down approach is also characteristic of the professionalized policy or practitioner perspective toward the ill and their problems. Even the most sensitive of policy thinkers does not escape this top-down perspective, often expressed in administrative, economic, and political terms (see, for instance, La Porte and Rubin, 1979; Meltzer, Farrow, and Richman, 1981). They fail to follow through as thoroughly as they might on their insights into the fateful situations and difficult work of the chronically ill, and, for that matter, on their knowledge of the inadequacies of health services and health personnel (see Vladeck, 1984). The language of many professionals shows the basic stance. There are people who "deliver" health care and people who "receive" health care. Sometimes health professionals talk about "consumers" and "providers," thinking about health services in market or even industrial terms. Clients and caretakers are supposed—or at least hoped—to act rationally and sensibly. Appropriate behavior includes their adhering to regimens faithfully, monitoring themselves or the ill person carefully, and reporting accurately to responsible practitioners. All of this presumably makes sense to most professionals, as it does, in part, to many clients. Yet it is far from the whole story. Laypeople see the regimens, services, practitioners, and so on as fitting or not fitting into the flow of illness-affected life (Corbin and Strauss, 1985, 1988). There is not necessarily a conflict between lay and professional views, but they are certainly not mirror images of each other.

One probable consequence is the professionals' inevitable piecemeal approach to the endemic problems of the chronically ill. Practitioners at clinics or physicians' offices or who visit the ill in their homes see many of them, but can see individuals only at intervals. They must necessarily monitor or assess ill people in their current state only. The temporal perspective of the ill person and kin is quite otherwise. Moreover, the problems of the ill and their kin are unquestionably theirs; they are not the problems of aggregates of ill persons, as the policy researchers and advocates are almost always likely to consider them owing to the very nature of policy research and advocacy. Also, as we have indicated, professionals are likely to see these problems from the standpoint of their own specialties and professional positions, however broad a perspective they have on chronic illness issues. Indeed, it is striking how specialized the literature that they tend to cite is, whether they are medical sociologists (Conrad, 1987), social worker–gerontologists (Brody, 1987), economists (Fein, 1986), or political scientists (Vladeck, 1983) with an eye on the pertinent governmental legislation. And, it is rare to find in the literature written by these otherwise astute critics as candid a statement as the following: "We are going to have to find better ways of making our care system more responsible to the expressed and implicit desires of clients and informal caretakers. How to do this in a systematic way is not something about which I have a lot to say" (Vladeck, 1983, p. 3).

The prevailing acute care approach to illness has proven to be inadequate to the task of providing care for the chronically ill. Strong criticisms of the acute care perspective and proposals for reform have been made by many critics, especially those professionally involved with rehabilitation or gerontology. Their suggestions, however, also suffer from a number of weaknesses, in part because of the inevitable difference between the professional attitude of the critics toward the ill and the concerns of the ill and their families themselves.

TWO

* * * * *

The Lives of
Chronically Ill People
and Their Families

In Part Two, we note that chronic illness consists of several very different phases, each requiring different types of care. Then we present case studies that illustrate these phases and that highlight the inadequacies of our health care system in addressing the problems encountered in these phases.

Chapter Five presents our theoretical framework or model for thinking about chronic illness and its related policy issues. This trajectory model emphasizes such matters as home care, quality of life, the lifelong work entailed in the management of illness, the several phases of illness, and the interplay of illness management and other forms of daily work. The concept of illness phase is especially important.

In Chapter Six, we discuss the recovery and rehabilitation, or comeback, phases of illness. They are not well served by the health care system when they last longer than a few months. Yet they present many psychological, social, and even clinical problems to the ill and their families. The cases in this chapter reflect the acute care orientation of physicians and the health care system in general and how it fails to serve people at home during comeback phases.

Chapter Seven discusses stable phases. Maintaining a stable physical state requires careful management by the ill and a spouse or other intimate. Management rests on effective and durable work arrangements. The case illustrations in this chapter show that the health care system serves the ill during stable phases only in the strictly clinical sense. There are gaps in accessibility to and availability of nonclinical services that affect the present and future stability of ill persons.

Chapter Eight discusses unstable phases of illness. Care of the ill during periods of instability is not wholly a matter of medical management. Our case illustrations suggest gaps in the health care system in relation to unstable phases of illness. Services that actually exist fail to reach many of the destabilized, and other services do not exist for long-term periods of instability.

Chapter Nine discusses deterioration. Along with acute phases, deterioration is what the health care system is most concerned with, as are the practitioners who work to prevent it or slow it down. Our cases are pertinent to policy considerations. They point up the gaps in service, especially in counseling and guidance, as well as some of the more drastic consequences—financial, psychological, and social—of government funding practices as well as of private insurance funding.

5

∗ ∗ ∗ ∗ ∗

Understanding
What It Means
to Be Chronically Ill

The perspectives of even the most perceptive and sensitive advocates of long-term care are probably informed with some degree of intellectualization. This leads them to see problems and issues piecemeal and from the top down, and to see ill people as an aggregate rather than as individuals with personal histories. Our own perspective is no exception, since we are also professionals: one of us is a nurse and the other is a sociologist. Yet the nature of our training and research has allowed us to capture much of the nonintellectualized, grass-roots experiences of the ill and their intimates, who experience their illness as part of their life as a whole. These experiences and our interpretations of them will be presented in the next chapters.

These interpretations, along with many years of research with the chronically ill, have led to and are in turn guided by a theoretical framework. The genesis of this framework, or model, goes back to the late 1960s. The senior author of this book, while studying how dying patients were given care by hospital staffs, realized that the overwhelming proportion of patients, whether dying or not, were chronically ill. He focused his next research efforts on discovering, through interviews and field observations, what the experiences were of the chronically ill and their helpers, both at home and in hospitals. Over the years he, his students, and interested colleagues have developed a set of theoretical interpretations about the medical, psychological, and organizational aspects of managing chronic illness. Their initial formulation provided the theoretical scheme presented in *Chronic Illness and the Quality of Life* (Strauss and Glaser, 1975).

The framework presented and used throughout this book is designed to supplement—not to supplant—health workers' thinking about the chronically ill and their problems. As Vladeck (1984, p. 7) has stated, long-term care should be continuous, flexible, responsive to what the ill require, and respectful of the ill and their families. The perplexing problem is how specifically to attain these goals. A large part of the answer is contained in the plethora of reform suggestions that were touched on in the last chapter. However, we also believe that to attain these goals, we must plan and institute health policies with a fuller awareness that the services offered the ill must take into account the considerations spelled out in our theoretical framework.

The Trajectory Model

This theoretical framework supports what we term a *trajectory model,* which can be expressed as a series of assertions.

1. Home is the central site—the major workplace—where lifelong illness is managed on a daily basis.

2. The major concern of the ill and their families is not merely nor primarily managing an illness, but maintaining the *quality of life,* as defined specifically by them, despite the illness.

3. Lifelong illness requires lifelong work to control its course, manage its symptoms, and live with the resulting disability. At home, the work is principally done by the ill themselves, if possible, and by family members, abetted perhaps by agency or purchased services. In health facilities, the work is done primarily by the staff, although even here patients do their share of the work.

4. As noted earlier, any course of illness will proceed through one or more of several phases.

5. Each of these phases calls for different kinds or combinations of work in different proportions by all participants: that is, work varies with the phase of the illness. The work by hospital staffs is addressed chiefly to acute phases of illness and to reparative surgery. Work at clinics and in physicians' offices is done mainly by physicians and nurses and mostly combines management of deteriorating phases with maintenance of some level of stability, but also includes work during the immediate posthospital medical recovery phase.

6. At home, there is an interplay of three major types of work: the work of managing illness; the everyday work of keeping a household and life in general going; and "biographical work"—the work associated with maintaining one's mental and psychological concerns as one would like them to be despite the impact of the illness and its management. This work is done chiefly by the ill and their families.

7. Within the context of home and family life, the central feature of illness management is the establishment and maintenance of arrangements. These arrangements enable the illness work to be more or less effective. Most arrangements involve organizing the time and effort of the ill person in conjunction with those of family members, and sometimes those of relatives, friends, and neighbors.

8. These arrangements are almost always revised and reorganized in accordance with changes in illness phase. Various life contingencies will also force rearrangements.

9. Maintaining these necessary arrangements, and making workable rearrangements, for carrying out the three types of work are continuous.

10. The work of health practitioners feeds into this continual and daily work. This work is frequently essential. Once the patient has returned from the hospital, however, he or she is thrown back on making or revising the arrangements necessary for carrying out regimens, visits to health facilities, and incorporating agency services into daily life. In short, the work of health practitioners is usually very much a part of the overall illness management, but it is only a part.

11. Its effectiveness in relation to long-term management depends not only on its technical efficiency and quality, but on

how well it supplements and is incorporated into the ongoing management work of the ill and their families.

12. Hence, a major and difficult practitioner and policy issue concerns the articulation of family and professional efforts at illness management. (In the literature, this is termed "informal and formal services," which connotes an emphasis on professional efforts.)

13. To break out of the prevailing medical-clinical perspective on chronic illness, and to capture the cumulative implications of the above points, health practitioners and those concerned with health policy should think in terms of the concept of illness trajectory. This term refers not only to a course of illness, but to the work of all participants involved in controlling and shaping that set of physiological events. It also refers to the impact of that work and the evolving relationships among the workers. So defined, the trajectory encompasses physiological events as well as the work of every participant, the work relationships, the changing work patterns, and the arrangements that are made to carry out the work in the face of changing illness phases and life's contingencies—all in the service of some conception of quality of life (Corbin and Strauss, 1988).

14. The implications of this trajectory model for health policy and practice include the following: (1) It should be recognized that with the currently incurable illnesses, efforts at health care should pertain to quality-of-life as well as strictly medical considerations. (2) Home should be regarded as the central workplace, and the families of the ill as key members in managing the illnesses, along with the health professionals. (3) The tremendous imbalance of funding and other resources between health facilities (especially the hospitals) and home care should be corrected. (4) Clinical (medical) services offered to the ill should be greatly supplemented by other types of services, including housekeeping, supportive caretaking, and various types of counseling (informational, psychological, marital, sexual, financial, legal, and so on). (5) Most of all, services should be sensitively and sensibly tailored both to changes in illness phase and to what the ill and their families can incorporate into their own continuing arrangements.

Critics of the current health care system will generally

recognize that this trajectory model implies some of the same correctives that can be found in the literature. However, professional perspectives (and often those of the gerontologists) lead to somewhat less radical critiques. Models that emphasize "patient/family responsibilities," matching professional services with "patients' needs," and even something as close to the trajectory model as a "client-based service model" do not grasp the fuller implications of what chronic illness prevalence means either for the health services or for the ill and their families themselves. As we have suggested earlier, an intellectualized perspective on health care is still dominant. Close listening to the ill themselves leads to a more grass-roots approach that nevertheless recognizes the crucial roles of health professionals and legislative and other experts in the total division of labor.

Trajectory is the central concept of the theoretical framework that lies behind this health policy model. It represents a social science approach to thinking about chronic illness, rather than the usual medical/nursing one. This concept focuses on the active role that persons play in shaping the course of an illness. This course is shaped not only by the nature of an illness and an ill person's unique response to it but also through actions taken by health personnel, the ill themselves, their spouses, and whoever else is involved in its management. Ultimately, however, it is the ill, their marital partners, and other intimates who carry out the day-to-day work involved in illness management, who work out the problems accompanying that work, and who in the end are most affected by the consequences of the illness and illness work.

In sum, the term *trajectory* captures aspects of the temporal phases of the illness, the work, the interplay of workers, and the nonmedical features of management along with relevant medical ones. It captures aspects of the experiences of everyone involved in the management drama, experiences that are anxious, puzzling, painful, as well as those on the brighter side. In some sense, illness is more or less fateful. The trajectory concept adds the aspect of fatefulness, of "undergoing and doing" (Dewey, 1934, p. 44), to what medical people call "treatment plans or programs" (Corbin and Strauss, 1988, p. 32).

This organizing concept has a set of related concepts that are vitally important for understanding what is involved in the management of an incurable illness. This is true whether the management is done at home or at health facilities. These concepts are particularly important for understanding the experiences of the ill and their intimates as those experiences are reflected in the cases presented in the next chapters.

Phases. People experience incurable illness—even a mild or generally stable one—as a series of phases. Sometimes the illness is *acute,* and may necessitate hospitalization. After such acute periods, the ill must recover physiologically. Recovery, or *comeback,* is both physiological and psychological; physiological recovery may be slow or incomplete and so create psychological and social problems. This phase, ideally, leads to a period of physiological or at least symptomatic *stability.* Some people also may experience periods of *instability* during which the disease or its symptoms cause their condition to fluctuate wildly. The complex phase commonly known as *deterioration,* in which the ill person's condition worsens, in turn may lead to a *dying* phase of varying duration. The cases described in the next chapters will illustrate some of the variants and subtleties of these six phases. Life for the ill and their families can be very different from one phase of an illness to the next. These phases can be more fully understood not simply as medical phenomena but as involving both work and biographical experiences.

Work. An illness is not just experienced as part of one's life; it must also be managed. Management requires work. At health facilities, the work is done by practitioners; at home, the ill themselves do the work, perhaps assisted by marital partners, intimates, other family members, caretakers, friends, neighbors, and health professionals (see, for instance, Gerhardt and Brieskorn-Zinke, 1986; De Mille, 1981; Labrie, 1986; Locker, 1983; Speedling, 1982; Schneider and Conrad, 1983; Strauss and Glaser, 1975).

The most obvious work involves following a regimen. When its tasks require little time, energy, or thought, the work is minimal. When the reverse is true, work can be onerous and even exhausting. The ill and their helpers, as the following case studies will show, perform several types of work. All types share a couple of general features, however. First, managing an illness and its symptoms or a disability is embedded in a context of ongoing daily life, in which everyday work (housekeeping, child rearing, earning a living) must go on. Second, illness work may intrude on other activities. Aside from the intrusiveness of symptoms, the treatment itself may be a disturbing factor for the entire family (Massie and Massie, 1973).

Work of Each Phase. The specifics of illness work, in kind and amount, usually vary by the phase of illness. During a diabetic crisis, for example, the work is immediately crucial; it must be done speedily and done right. This crisis work is quite different from the procedural tasks characteristic of the prevailing stable phases. After many decades of diabetes, deterioration may require yet other kinds of work.

Resources for Each Phase. The kind and amount of the resources needed for carrying out the required illness work also vary by illness phase. This leads to additional complexities in the nature of illness work. Resources—strength, energy, adequate savings—often are not on hand and may have to be sought out, discovered, bargained for, or purchased. Once obtained, resources have to be replenished or replaced if they fail. Consequently, when the illness moves into another phase, the cluster of resources previously adequate may now be inadequate (not enough or good enough) or inappropriate (doesn't fit, or is no longer needed). This shifting resource requirement is like the changing need of a family for a particular house: the house that fits a family's requirements exactly at a given time may, as the family increases, its children grow older, and its interests change, later become inadequate or inappropriate to the family's changed size, character, or interests.

This changing need for resources is generally recognized by sensitive health practitioners. Often they can help to solve resource deficits, but frequently the health care system itself blocks this possibility. Also, sometimes there are miniphases within the longer arc of a phase, such as days of relative stability in a phase of deterioration, or a rapid series of permanent drops in a generally deteriorating physical condition. During these short periods, the work that is required will vary; the appropriate resources for doing the work will also vary.

Arrangements. A key concept in our theoretical scheme is that of "arrangements." In order to get the illness work accomplished, all kinds of arrangements have to be instituted and maintained. The arrangements also have to be revised for every major shift in phase, and sometimes even for minor shifts. Arrangements pertain not only to illness management but also to what has to be done to make that management possible. For example, a person partly disabled by illness must not only manage the symptoms of the illness but also devise ways to perform all the ordinary tasks of living. For this reason, the ill and their intimates develop domestic, kin, friendship, and neighborhood arrangements. Even participants in self-help groups (Denzin, 1986; Maines, 1984) make such arrangements to support their routine tasks and strategies for handling their key problems. As we have written in a previous publication (Strauss and others, 1984, p. 17):

> Strategies for coping with key problems call for certain kinds of *organizational* or *family arrangements*. People's efforts must be coordinated—with all the understandings and agreements that necessitates. Thus disabled patients have standing arrangements with neighbors and friends who do their grocery shopping for them. The parents of diabetic children need to coach neighbors in reading the signs of oncoming coma as well as to warn them against allowing the child to have sweets while at their homes. A man with a cardiac condition and his wife may reach an agreement—perhaps only after much persuasion by her—that when she senses his oncoming fatigue before he does, she will warn him; otherwise he may

suddenly and embarrassingly run out of energy.
Clearly, to establish and maintain such necessary
arrangements may require not only much trust and
considerable interactional skill but also financial,
medical, and family resources. If any of those are
lacking, the arrangements may never be properly
instituted or may collapse. In any case, important
consequences—for both the patient and his or her
family—flow from how he or she and they have
organized their efforts so as to handle key problems.

Some of these arrangements call for or evolve into relationships
with certain persons "who act as various kinds of *agents*. Thus . . .
people . . . act as *rescuing* agents . . . or as *protective agents* (accompanying an epileptic person so that if she begins to fall she
can be eased to the ground), or as *assisting agents* (helping with
a regimen), or as *control* agents (making the patient stay with
her regimen), and so on" (p. 17).

Biographical Concerns and Biographical Work. Every
perceptive home care practitioner is sensitive to the psychological
aspects of clients' problems and takes them into account when
offering care. These psychological aspects must also be built into
a theoretical framework that can be pertinent to long-term care
policy. A severe chronic illness, even during its stable phases,
can destructively affect the biographies of the ill, their intimates,
and their families (Bury, 1982; Davis, 1973; Kutner, 1987). Personal and family suffering can be generated by the strains of
prolonged illness, the work it requires, and the changes in household, job, and social relationships it brings about. From our
research, it has become clear to us that disturbed biographical
concerns result in a tremendous amount of what we term *biographical work*. People have to work at solving problems of identity—their own and often that of their intimates. They must find
new goals in life or new ways to achieve old ones (Charmaz,
1983, 1987; Maines, 1983). The concept of biographical work
is more elusive than that of trajectory phase, work, or arrange-

ments, but it refers to a phenomenon of great importance. A key question for the practitioner—as well as for those doing the work—is just what kind of biographical work is going on and in reference to what biographical problem. How the work is done and its measure of success will inevitably affect the specifics of illness management, including who does what tasks, how, and how much. We shall have much to say about this topic in the next chapters.

Articulation. To put together all the arrangements, resources, interactional strategies, agents, tasks, and action can be difficult. Keeping all of these constituents together is even more difficult than initiating them, given unexpected medical contingencies as well as the contingencies of just plain living. When the management mechanisms begin to go out of kilter, this relatively silent process of putting and keeping together becomes more visible. It is an enduring aspect of the lives and experiences of the chronically ill and those around them (Corbin and Strauss, 1988).

These, then, are the main elements of the theoretical framework that guides our policy-oriented commentaries on the illustrative cases in the next chapters. Our theoretical concepts and their implications are grounded primarily not in clinical experience but in our years of listening to, querying, and observing the diverse actors who seek to keep illnesses under control in the hospital and to juggle management at home within the context of both immediate and long-term personal and familial considerations.

Note on Case Illustrations

The picture of the health care system sketched in the previous chapters, and the critics' views of its performance in long-term care, are after all a picture painted by people who are very aware of the system's overall structure and functioning. They see and judge it on the basis of a great deal of knowledge. By contrast, the people who encounter aspects of the system when they or their family members become chronically ill see the system as it works or does not work for *themselves*. However, they can scarcely encounter all of its features. Often, they do not conceive of it as a system. They only see certain services as relating to themselves and their problems. Also, even after years of illness, they are usually unaware of other services of which they could have availed themselves.

In the next chapters, we present case studies of several chronically ill persons, living alone, with spouses or partners, or with families. In these cases, all the illness phases except the hospitalized acute phase are illustrated in detail. All but three cases are précis of interviews done for a research project directed at understanding the work done by the chronically ill and their marital partners in managing illness. The interviews and the interviewees are described in Corbin and Strauss (1988). That monograph also elaborates on the theoretical framework detailed in Chapter Five. Both the descriptions of the cases and our commentaries are designed to bring out the reality of how the health services fit into the lives of the ill and their families. Sometimes these services are seen as crucial, sometimes as peripheral, albeit necessary in some regard. Sometimes these people's use of the health care system may seem relatively inefficient. If so, the cases also suggest what is wrong with current arrangements, what keeps available services from being suggested or offered to those who need them.

Our commentaries on the cases also underline two other points. First, the cases show us something of what is lacking in the health care system, supplying illustrative detail for the more abstract, bare-bones criticism made by long-term care practitioners and people who write about policy. Second, the cases illustrate vividly the kinds of resources the ill and their intimates actually draw upon, how they stay afloat—or sink— when living with severe chronic illness. Policymakers and practitioners can learn a great deal about how the ill manage their illnesses while at the same time striving for some quality of life, as they define it. The information drawn from our cases will be supplemented and fortified by occasional material from our other research. *We do not base our policy-practitioner recommendations here or in later chapters solely on these particular case illustrations.*

The people who appear in the case illustrations were among the sixty couples and several single persons whom we interviewed in our last study (Corbin and Strauss, 1988). All but three of the ill men and women were living as couples with spouses or, in one instance, with a partner of the same sex. In a few instances, both partners were ill. Their illnesses included cardiac disease, diabetes, cancer, arthritis, asthma, Alzheimer's disease, multiple sclerosis, Parkinson's disease, schizophrenia, and illnesses precipitated by quadriplegia. Some of the ill suffered from two or more conditions. Each of the different illness phases except the hospitalized acute phase will be illustrated in detail by our case narratives. The working relationships of the partners are variously and to some degree collaborative, cooperative, conflicted, or even symbiotic.

These people are recognizably working class, lower middle class, and middle class, as judged by their life-styles, educational levels, and economic statuses. They represent both blue-collar and so-called "middle" America. They are neither at the bottom nor the top of America's socioeconomic ladder. They are not poor or destitute; on the other hand, they are not wealthy or very affluent. Because most of them are in their middle or later years, however, they tend to have more financial resources than if they were younger. While some are on Medicare, none are on welfare, nor will they be eligible for Medicaid until they run through all of their savings. At worst, these people can be rendered destitute by catastrophic or long-term illness.

Some of the people who appear in the case illustrations are managing in the face of incurable illnesses; others are barely hanging in there. Yet even those who are managing are lacking one or more resources that would enhance their management and most certainly improve the quality of their lives. One would expect these average Americans to have the resources needed to do well despite illness. After all, they are educated and have achieved desired standards of living. But because chronic illnesses are debilitating and long-term, they wear down even the middle class physically, psychologically, and financially. It is precisely for this reason that we have chosen these people to use as case illustrations. If they are having difficulties in managing, think of how much more difficult it is for those who have fewer resources, or who are physically fragile yet live alone.

Some of the interpretations and implications of such cases were made in a somewhat different form by one of the authors as early as 1975 (Strauss and Glaser, 1975). This underlines how little basic change there has been in the past decade in thinking about the policy and practice implications of chronic illness. Certainly there are more services for the chronically ill, a greater concern (especially for the sick elderly), and some attitudinal changes among health professionals; but very little seems to have changed in the lives of the ill themselves—exemplified by our case illustrations and other people whom we have studied—as they struggle to stay afloat in the face of severe chronic illness.

6

★ ★ ★ ★ ★

Recovering from
a Medical Crisis

The comeback phase of illness, commonly referred to as recovery or as a period of rehabilitation, is recognized to be of great clinical importance. Extensive rehabilitation services have been set up for certain kinds of illness, especially for sufferers from strokes and spinal cord injuries. Yet the health care system does not address the problems of most of those who must struggle through recovery periods of any length. In this chapter, we bring out the issues involved with long and difficult recoveries, especially their nonclinical aspects.

A comeback involves an uphill course, following an acute episode of a chronic illness, to what is perceived as a satisfactory way of living within the limits imposed by the illness itself. At any point throughout lifelong illness, a comeback may involve attempts to regain salient aspects of oneself that were lost during a severe acute phase (such as a severe stroke or heart attack). The road back may then be long and difficult, marked by small setbacks, some marked improvement, and plateaus of indefinite duration. Moreover, indicators of progress may be extremely ambiguous. In a physical sense, comebacks may of course be only partial. Bodily and social actions, as well as personal accomplishments, may fall short of past ones.

Three general processes seem to be involved in any comeback. First, there is "mending," the process of physical healing. Second, there is the "stretching of physical limitations," pushing the body to the boundaries of its current abilities. This may increase body performance as well as hasten or improve its mending. Rehabilitative services, of course, are designed to do this. Third, there is "reknitting," the ill person's putting his or her biography back together again, within the actual and perceived limitations of body and social performance.

These three processes are usually not sequential but are simultaneous. Yet in the transition days when an acute period is moving into recovery, attention is still focused on the management of acute physical distress and its symptoms. The concerns of physicians, nurses, family, and the ill person center on necessary illness work and immediate questions about the illness. What course will it take in the near future? What clinical interventions will be necessary to put the ill person on the road to recovery? What will be the residual effects, if any, and how can they be prevented? Since the illness itself is in focus, biographical concerns, and often rehabilitation also, are relegated temporarily to secondary status. When the immediate acute period is over and the physical condition is relatively stable, the ill person either returns to normal living or faces residual body limitations and what those mean for his or her life.

Progress along the comeback trail is marked by statements such as "Today I was able to feed myself," "Now I can walk up this slight incline without angina," or "Finally I taught my first class, using my newly learned mode of speech." These progress statements can be clear or ambiguous. Often they serve as confidence boosters, which help one put the pieces of life back together and increase one's motivation to continue to mend and to stretch limitations. By the same token, setbacks can act as confidence smashers, which can sometimes halt efforts to come back permanently.

If the comeback period follows on a severe or critical acute phase, then usually the ill person and often his or her intimates will ask a series of questions. These questions are colored by uncertainty about the ill person's ability to perform socially and physically. For instance:

1. How reversible is this illness? How far back will or can I go? Which of my previous activities will I be able to pursue?
2. How quickly will I come back: partially? most of the way? all the way?
3. How long will I remain on the present plateau before moving upward? How soon will I really know?
4. Can my own actions affect the amount or rate of my comeback? What actions will improve my chances: following the prescribed regimen? praying? something else? How much of this must I do and for how long?
5. What about hourly, daily, or weekly fluctuations in my functioning? How much of that will always be part of my life? When will I know for sure?

Biographical considerations aside, the basic components of a comeback—resources, work, and arrangements—are the same whether the period is complicated and of long duration or relatively simple and short. The physician is likely to prescribe a regimen and, for a few illnesses, rehabilitation services also. Regimens may entail much work and require the making of arrangements if assistance from others is needed, or if a spouse's cooperation is requisite, as when a wife must alter her cooking style to suit her husband's low-salt diet. The physician may also prescribe "rest," or use phrases like "take it easy for a while" and "don't climb those stairs too often." However these injunctions are interpreted once the ill are back home, they are likely to require rearrangements of the marital or family division of labor. Furthermore, if the spouse is overburdened or the ill person is living alone, they will call on friends and kin or obtain the services of home care agencies, if those are available. At the very least, someone else may have to shop for groceries and take out the garbage.

Another major and continuing task during comebacks is the necessity to monitor the bodily signs of the ill. If they do not wish or are not able to do it themselves, others are drawn into the monitoring—and also sometimes into reproving or coaching the ill person, using phrases like "you look tired now" or "you should stop and rest whenever you feel like this and not wait so long." Other people are often needed as motivating agents—to urge the ill to persist with painful, boring, or seemingly useless regimens, to keep up flagging spirits and faith in attaining at least some measure of recovery.

For comeback into the wider world, job arrangements may be needed. Sick leave arrangements have to be requested or bargained for if the organizational arrangements do not exist. If the spouse or other caretaker has a paid job but is needed at home, then he or she may have to make similar arrangements. If the ill person owns a business or is an executive, complicated organizational arrangements will have to be made. There are also the bothersome and sometimes anxiety-provoking tasks of keeping track of and paying medical bills during this period.

To find the necessary resources, to make and maintain the necessary arrangements, to keep everything going, may or may not be difficult in any particular comeback period. This depends on the disability of the ill, the resources at hand, and so on. Yet the difference between a brief comeback period and one that is prolonged is striking, as well as relevant for policy-making. A long recovery period usually is more difficult both clinically and psychologically. Inevitably, the problems of maintaining resources and sustaining the supporting arrangements also increase, sometimes frighteningly. Because the health care system is organized around acute care and the practitioners operate in terms of that, however, the institutional services available to recovering patients tend to be limited in duration and often in scope. The implications of this situation will be discussed later in this chapter.

Laura: An Acute, Short-Term Comeback

Laura is a single woman who lives alone in a small apartment. She is in her late forties, in excellent physical shape, and an expert jogger. Her experiences exemplify the early weeks of a comeback from an acute problem that involved no chronic complications. We use this acute case because it clearly shows the kinds of arrangements that need to be made, especially if one is single, and even if the disability is not serious enough to deplete one's energy, keep one bedridden, or leave one dizzy or slow in mental responses. Laura's problem was simply one of relative immobility, but this considerably affected her life for several weeks. Her case also suggests the particular weaknesses of the health care system in relation to short comeback periods.

Returning to her apartment one morning from grocery shopping, Laura slipped on a newly waxed floor and broke her right leg. She remained in the hospital for over ten days, an unexpectedly long period of time, because of the great amount of tissue damage accompanying the fracture. She was told the leg would be back to normal in about six months. Before she returned home, she borrowed crutches from a cousin. She also arranged with a friend to be driven home from the hospital. She had figured out the problem of navigating a flight of stairs, and her friend helped her to mount them. She negotiated with the landlord to have the handrail strengthened thereafter in order to support her careful maneuvering down and up the stairs. She also worked out with a hospital-assigned physical therapist how best to move up and down the stairs, after she discovered that the carpet was uneven and so presented certain problems not foreseen by the physical therapist.

Laura was strong enough and unimpeded enough by her disabled leg to use a walker or crutches to move around the apartment, to get in and out of bed, and eventually to go out of her apartment or on occasional drives with friends. She had no difficulty with her personal care, although she had to purchase a special bath chair. She was even able to cook, but found it difficult and impractical to carry crockery and food from her tiny kitchen to the living-room table. All of these activities were managed without making special arrangements with other people. For housekeeping chores, however, since she had no spouse or companion to help, she had to make arrangements with friends. Fortunately, her many friends were cooperative and found time to take turns doing tasks. Their chief duties were to make her bed, take the laundry to and from the cleaner's, carry the garbage can, bring in and send out the day's mail, and above all to shop for groceries. Friends with autos made it easier and cheaper to visit the physician for weekly checkups on the healing of her fracture.

The arrangements that Laura was able to make concerning her job were also essential to her comeback. She was a university professor of long standing. Some of the same friends who helped with household chores were departmental colleagues and could also assist here. The first couple of weeks after her accident were covered by sick leave (otherwise she would have had to request it). When she returned to work, she was driven to and from work by colleagues and friends. They also helped in her first days back at work, seeing that doors were opened for her. Luckily, the campus was relatively flat, so that she could use a wheelchair to move from building to building. This allowed Laura to teach all of her assigned classes; otherwise she might have had to make arrangements for that contingency, too.

Five weeks down the comeback trail, everyone was well set in their routines. Laura was now able to take her laundry to and from the cleaner's herself. On the advice of the physical therapist, she rode her stationary bicycle faithfully. Recently, she had been disturbed because her disabled leg had lost considerable weight and she had been told that it would take some months to recoup the muscle tone. A friend suggested she ask her physician whether it would be useful to visit a sports therapist for counseling and exercises. The physician approved, and the sports therapist has turned out to have useful ideas.

Looking forward to the next weeks of recuperation, Laura now sees no unsolvable problems. Thinking about living alone, her age, and the years ahead, however, she has begun to imagine what would have happened to her if an accident or an illness had left her disabled or debilitated for a much longer period. For instance, her health insurance pays for only one hundred home visiting services. What would have happened if she had had to use such services for longer than that?

She now understands that the use of an informal network of friends takes judicious and delicate maneuvering, requiring considerable managerial skill. Friends were willing to help, but sometimes found it difficult to schedule their visits, or were out of town, or became sick themselves. Consequently, they were somewhat unreliable helpers, despite their willingness to make Laura's life easier. Furthermore, they could not have been depended on heavily for more than a few months. Yet they were a crucial factor in her comeback. If she had had to do more chores herself, she might have suffered setbacks, possibly severe ones.

Friends were essential to another major feature of her life and her economic survival: getting her to and from her job. Because she works at a university, she would not have lost her job if her forced absence had exceeded her official amount of sick leave, but there are limits to the patience of an organization, and of colleagues. Working was essential to her sense of accomplishment, of being her old self again. Just to get back to it is a marker of progress toward full recovery and a normal existence. Friends were very helpful too in lightening her depression at the unexpected slowness of her initial steps in physical recovery.

Laura's case thus underlines both the strengths and weaknesses of our health care system. The system is strong in the medical care given during acute and immediate postacute periods, but weak in the slight nonclinical but important support during the weeks thereafter. If her disability had turned out to be chronic (as it almost did), the weakness of the system would have become even more evident.

Mrs. Scully: Few or No
Rehabilitation Services, Little Comeback

Comebacks ordinarily begin in the hospital, if the patient is fortunate enough to be at the right hospital, on the right ward, with thoughtful and effective comeback agents. These agents are a knowledgeable attending physician, alert and sensitive nurses, and, if necessary, a knowledgeable social worker, efficient physical and recreational therapists, and perhaps sexual and psychological counselors. A recovery phase may even begin in an ICU. Patients with Guillain-Barré Syndrome, for example, begin rehabilitation in the hospital. About 85 percent of these patients recover to normal functioning, only about 5 per-

cent having significant neurological impairment. Hospital personnel can maintain flexibility of joints and muscular tone and
prevent residual effects through physiotherapy. Since physical
recovery takes from two weeks to three years, however, the personnel cannot reply with certainty to patients' specific questions
about their recovery. Consequently, staffs believe that educating
patients and families about the disease is especially necessary
throughout this portion of the recovery period, particularly
because the patient's psychological reactions to the slow process of recovery may be intense. Patients who have suffered
strokes or accidents that have left them paraplegic or quadriplegic
are also moved into the rehabilitation phase while they are still
hospitalized.

Sometimes, however, even stroke victims fall between institutional cracks, getting few or ineffective rehabilitation services. Mrs. Scully, housed in a nursing home, is a patient who
seemed never to have been fortunate enough even to begin much
of a comeback. When we met her, she seemed out of place in
the nursing home. She was fairly alert, and only in her late fifties. She had suffered a stroke several years before. Her condition seemed bad, but not extremely so. We wondered at first
why she had not been able to receive the kind of rehabilitative
services that might at least have enabled her to avoid her sad fate.

Despite her fairly high level of education and her middle-
income status at the time of the stroke, several conditions mitigated against her receiving the extensive rehabilitation services
that her physical condition warranted. Mrs. Scully was a widow
living alone, her son living elsewhere. There was no spouse or
family to research services that were available for improving
her chances of recovery. Apparently her son did not play this
role either. We do not know if her neurologist faded out of the
picture quickly after the acute phase was over, or if there were
other factors that blocked or impeded the use of rehabilitative
services. Possibly, as sometimes happens, a rehabilitation staff
decided after a time that she was hopeless or insufficiently moti-
vated. They may even have given her short shrift after a quick
assessment as not a "good bet" (Kaufman and Becker, 1986).
After all, there are many patients, and some are more likely

to "deserve" the staff's strenuous efforts on their behalf than others.

For stroke sufferers like Mrs. Scully, living alone is a disaster. Either they cannot manage by themselves, or others believe they cannot. Consequently, they often end up in nursing homes, like many highly deteriorated single persons—the fragile elderly or people in the later stages of Alzheimer's disease. Yet sometimes people like Mrs. Scully ought not to be in nursing homes at all. Appropriate rehabilitation services might have helped them come back enough to stay out of nursing homes, or they might at least be maintained in more humane settings. Nursing homes are generally thought of as repositories for extremely deteriorated or dying patients, the institutional graveyards of people who never were given much chance for even a partial comeback.

These ill people have counterparts who are able to live at home because of caretaking spouses or other kin. These are stroke victims and other severely debilitated or disabled persons who may have had fairly successful comebacks and good rehabilitative services, but who later suffered one or more dispiriting major setbacks. In consequence, they and perhaps their caretakers too have given up. They simply lack the motivation to "go through all of that again." After all, a comeback is not necessarily an easy period to endure, nor are rehabilitative tasks free of pain or drain on energy. Besides, these ill people ask, "What will ensure that I will not relapse again?" It takes determined professionals to combat motivational collapses like those. Generally, therefore, these ill people languish at home. If they suffer from illnesses like arthritis, rheumatism, or cardiac disease, their lack of rehabilitative effort and even of exercise contributes to their quicker physical deterioration.

Among those who have never even had a chance at a comeback are those who have been discouraged from stretching their own limits or bothering with rehabilitative services. This happens when physicians decide the patient is too far gone (Kaufman and Becker, 1986) or when spouses tell their partners not to overexert themselves because they could bring on another heart attack. In one careful study, it was found that predominant among the "cardiac cripples" were those who had been discouraged from trying to come back by spouses and physicians; by employers who refused to continue their employment or rehire them; and by insurance companies, whose policies tend to discourage efforts that might lead to relapses (Reif, 1975b). As one rehabilitation expert notes: "Other clients find that they are forced into a sick role by their families. Families and even some health personnel do not always encourage a person, especially an older person, to adapt to the disability to the fullest possible extent. Doctors tell arthritics not to. walk, daughters tell their mothers with congestive heart failure (CHF) to rest 'because it's time to take it easy.' Bowe (1978) notes that recently disabled people end up with perceptions of diminished worth as human beings because of the impact of problems of daily living that come from disability, reduced social status, and decreased income. As self-concepts become damaged, aspirations are lowered and isolation increases, further handicapping the individual" (Schank, 1986, p. 363).

In short, some people do not have the luck even to be started on a genuine comeback; they are either discouraged from embarking on the trail or literally do not know how to find or get into the necessary rehabilitative services. This is so even when these services are available or there is money to pay for them. Sometimes it requires someone else—a professional, relative, friend, or acquaintance—to open up rehabilitative possibilities to the ill. Otherwise, it takes ability and energy to ferret out the possible options.

A woman of our acquaintance, whose husband had undergone brain surgery at a health maintenance organization (HMO) and suffered two or three convulsions thereafter, could get no reassurance or useful counsel from his neurologist or internist. Finally, in desperation, she telephoned a family survival center advertised on the local buses. At relatively little cost to her, this center did an extensive neurological assessment, complete with recommendations for speech and neurological therapy. Armed with this report, the furious wife accosted the HMO physicians, who agreed that these therapies might be useful and forthwith prescribed them. The HMO also paid for the additional services. Whether or not her husband improves or his deterioration is slowed is not the point. Rather, it is that this wife's persistence and intelligence allowed her to break through the health care system as she and her husband were experiencing it. The system itself, she believes, must be manipulated, otherwise no recovery would be possible for ill people like her husband.

Alfredo: A Good Outcome— Could It Have Been Better or Easier?

The next case illustrates several points at which health services might be much improved by thinking in terms of more subtle features of chronic illness. First, the case shows the kinds of arrangements that are typically made when the ill are lucky enough to have spouses and cooperative friends. Second, this case illustrates how people with certain illnesses are left essentially on their own to seek out relevant knowledge, discover pertinent resources, and make their own facilitating arrangements in order to foster their comebacks. Third, the case illustrates the genuinely biographical character of such comebacks; except in purely clinical ways, the ill may not connect with useful rehabilitation services. Perhaps this is so even with regard to clinical matters.

Alfredo had a myocardial infarction in 1972, from which he slowly recovered enough to resume normal activities. Eight years later he had congestive heart failure so severe that his cardiologist wondered silently if he would ever leave his house again. Alfredo did not learn of his cardiologist's opinion until four months later, when his comeback was well under way.

Since he, too, was a university professor, he was able to take sick leave from October to January. He then taught his usual research seminar at home for the remainder of the academic year. In fact, his cooperative colleagues relieved him of all other university duties until the following autumn, by which time his physical recovery was at least symptomatically good. In the first couple of months after his hospitalization, his experienced research team carried on without him, then arranged to meet weekly at his home for conferences; frequently, too, they reported in by phone. Doctoral students working under his direction also came for conferences at his home.

Just before he left the hospital, Alfredo was given a regimen and some instructions. His medication was partly new, partly the same. Now, however, he was also put on a low-salt diet, which a hospital dietician explained to him and his wife. The dietician also gave them a list of the sodium content of various foods, which they nervously studied. He was sent home with instructions to rent a respirator machine, and shown how to use one correctly by a respiratory therapist before leaving the hospital. It was suggested that he "posture" for the drainage of his lungs, which would also help his chronic bronchitis. He also had severe back pains, which his heavy and frequent coughing exacerbated. Together, these symptoms left him even further exhausted than he might have been otherwise, yet he was not being visited by rehabilitation personnel who might have recognized this and done something effective to counter it. Cardiac rehabilitation was available, but the cardiologist did not believe his patient's condition warranted it.

At home, the regimen was followed closely. Medicare and private health insurance paid for medications, equipment, and visits to physicians. The matter of diet provoked much anxiety for Alfredo's wife, who saw her cooking duties as crucial to his recovery. The dietary information given at the hospital had been brief and not reassuring. The couple made the usual experiments with making interesting, low-salt meals, and two friends who were nurses were helpful in suggesting low-salt recipes and cookbooks. One nurse friend also helped with the initial taking of daily blood pressure, since the readings were difficult for the wife to make. Nobody else had thought to help her. Eventually, the patient himself discovered, in a magazine published for the elderly, that self-reading pressure machines were available. No professional had told him this. His wife finally suggested to the chest specialist that her husband perhaps should take antibiotics for one week each month in order to cut down on his frequent and exhausting coughing. This suggestion was taken up and proved successful. However, the lessons on deep breathing given at the hospital by a respiratory therapist were only a partial success. Many months later the patient, entirely by himself, finally learned how to do his daily breathing exercises correctly. Once again, it was a nurse friend who was helpful in assessing that he had indeed learned to breathe correctly.

Alfredo and his wife had to institute a new division of labor in the housekeeping work. At first he abstained from doing any chores. Fortunately, she was able to manage almost everything necessary by cutting back drastically on her long-standing and important voluntary work. For the occasional heavy tasks, she called on the services of male friends. She made certain for many weeks that her husband was not alone in the house; she ordered groceries over the phone, had friends bring them, or had friends cover for her while she was shopping. While he was perfectly capable of managing his personal grooming, she insisted in the first days after hospitalization on entering the shower with him and soaping him so that his exertion would be minimal. She also kept a watchful eye on him, monitoring his physical appearance and his energy, suggesting that he rest when he looked tired and becoming expert at reading cues about the likelihood of his falling apart. (Again, one wonders what happens to people who live alone, without spouses or companions.)

Accompanying Alfredo's physical comeback were the usual psychological and biographical phenomena. For example, he became puzzled because his "mind was now working well," yet he could not walk more than a block outside without angina. He broached the subject to his cardiologist, who now confessed that perhaps this was as much walking as Alfredo would ever be able to do. Fortunately, Alfredo did not believe him. Nevertheless, he and his wife had to struggle internally with the prospect of his becoming a cardiac cripple. Without professional counseling, they worked through this biographical crisis. The physician's tentative prediction was proven in the next two or three months to be wrong, to everyone's relief. Alfredo's other biographical work centered on facing long plateaus and occasional small setbacks, and frustration over daily fluctuations of energy. Since energy is a basic condition for activity of any kind, fluctuations in energy made his life, for many months, somewhat unpredictable.

Alfredo was fortunate in having a wife who could be at home, cooperative friends and employer, and private health insurance. He was also fortunate in being able to make the necessary arrangements for services of various kinds that were useful and perhaps vital for his comeback. He and his wife were sent home from the hospital with some basic instructions about the regimen; these instructions, however, were not helpful until they were supplemented by the informed knowledge and suggestions of friends and by other information.

Alfredo's problem was made more complicated clinically because the cardiologist and the chest specialist, though physicians at the same hospital, were focusing on improving the patient's cardiac and respiratory functioning, respectively. He himself had to supplement their individual regimens in order to bring his cardiac and respiratory systems into harmony. Meanwhile, neither physician was concerned with his back problem; they considered that this condition was not seriously complicating his major clinical problems. Consequently, he had to do a certain amount of therapeutic coordination of all three of his physical conditions. Moreover, since he had no professional visiting services, nobody gave expert counsel for managing the reciprocal impacts of these three conditions.

Alfredo and his wife were also left on their own to handle the biographical issues that accompany such a long and problematic comeback. While professional medical management of such comebacks is usually handled competently, there is a failure to utilize available rehabilitative counseling services. Fortunately, the ill are often psychologically strong and astute enough to struggle through the biographical (and sometimes clinical) issues by themselves, or with the help of close kin or friends. Sometimes they have recourse to the services of psychiatrists and psychologists; if they are fortunate, they find a helpful counselor for any sexual problems that may have developed. Cardiac and other types of illness can cause sexual difficulties; it is not known to what extent physicians initiate conversation about this matter or refer patients to competent counselors when the patients broach the topic. Generally, the gulf between medical specialists and those who deal with psychological problems is wide; a sizable segment of acute care–oriented physicians may not especially value the services of the latter. Yet it is clear that biographical processes may considerably affect clinical processes.

Commentary

The basic policy issue raised by comeback phases is that they are not sufficiently serviced except when they are short. Even then, the rehabilitation aspects of most chronic illnesses are not covered unless they fall under legislatively mandated services for the physically disabled (such as those suffering from strokes and spinal-cord injuries). All but the shortest recoveries require many more services than they get in order to be successful. After acute episodes, therefore, some portion of the chronically ill regain very little of their former functioning, while others regain far less than they might. Even when there is total recovery, the process is much more difficult than it need be. Moreover, unsuccessful comebacks lead to more frequent acute episodes, requiring increased medical expenses and perhaps hospitalization; or they lead to more rapid and seemingly inexorable physical deterioration.

If we look specifically at speedy comebacks from illnesses not covered by the government's specialized rehabilitation services, we see that funds from federal, state, or private insurance sources are inadequate to support even these comebacks. The chronically ill must pay for such services themselves. Moreover, at most rehabilitation agencies and departments, the personnel tend to be far less focused on the chronically ill than on the physically disabled, for whom most services were originally instituted. As one informed rehabilitation specialist has noted, "Rehabilitation teams tend not to work with the chronically ill. Apparently the rehabilitation team does not fully recognize the need of the chronically ill for its services, even if the rehabilitation directors do acknowledge that restorative services for the chronically ill would improve quality of life" (Schank, 1986, p. 360).

A further impediment to the use of rehabilitation services is the acute care perspective of physicians, who either greatly undervalue these services or are so concentrated on guiding physiological recovery that they do not think about what the rehabilitation people term "activities of daily living" (ADLs). Only about half of the medical schools have rehabilitation in their curricula, and the subject is low on the scale of faculty and student interests (Kottke, 1980; Fowler, 1982). In schools of nursing, "the acute care model continues to be the primary emphasis" (Schank, 1986, p. 360).

If the focus is so much on acute care during speedy recoveries, consider the problem when a comeback takes six months, a year, two years, or longer. During the first months, only the beginning of a comeback is made by anyone who has been seriously ill, whether for the first time or again and again. It may take many weeks before basic activities—a job, housework—can be done. This is because the ill person still has insufficient energy or mobility, or perhaps can only work at a slower pace and for a shorter time. How long will the paid job be kept open? Who will pay for whatever home care services are needed? Who will pay for such a long period of rehabilitation services? A minority of Americans are fortunate enough to be eligible for Veterans Administration services; the remainder pay for those services themselves, at least after the first months of acute care, unless they are on welfare. How long will their savings hold out? Considering all other demands on the same money, for how long will the ill person and family think that their money should be used for such services? Furthermore, longer comebacks entail not only the rebuilding and retraining of physically impaired bodies but finding new jobs, deciding on new careers, and developing new directions for life.

The severity of illness has particular relevance for policy considerations. An acute episode with many physical and physiological residuals is likely to require continuing medical care over a long time. The ill person may also need or profit from various types of counseling: job, financial, psychological, marital, and sexual. Those who are experiencing less difficult physical recoveries might still profit from home services, job retraining opportunities, and counseling, in order to prevent relapses. Setbacks in physical condition may well occur after the early recovery period has been passed through and the patient is believed to be stabilized. In the immediate postrecovery period, too, there are likely to be fluctuations of condition. These need to be closely monitored and downward cycles prevented by careful professional assessment and quick action. Spouses and other intimates, of course, do this in their own fashion. The ill who live alone are therefore especially vulnerable to setbacks. Unfavorable home conditions also may lead to setbacks, as may the flagging motivation of the ill and their helpers.

When an illness is likely to be fatal, as is childhood cystic fibrosis, symptomatic fluctuations are intensely monitored by family members and, if need be, by professionals. This is true during comeback periods as well as long periods of stability. In nonfatal illnesses such as severe arthritis, by contrast, when fluctuations are so much a part of the illness, health professionals are less likely to think of them as more than temporary, expected moments in the recovery itself. ''It all takes time and there will be difficult moments.''

The foregoing add up to a set of striking gaps in the health care services available to the chronically ill during their comeback phase. Even when services are available, people do not necessarily get to them for the variety of reasons noted throughout this chapter. The services may also be inaccessible because this is one of the times when the bureaucratic structure of the agencies is difficult to penetrate by still-weak ill people and their helpers. The latter then are frequently overworked and overwrought. The services that do exist are not reaching those whom they should reach—and there are not nearly enough of them.

Nearly a decade ago, Verville (1979) criticized rehabilitation services for the physically disabled. His criticisms are equally applicable to the rehabilitative-restorative services for the chronically ill, although these are so vital to successful comebacks. Verville's observations have been summarized by Schank (1986, p. 360), thus: (1) The disabled are not encouraged to become rehabilitated. (2) Financing of rehabilitation care is inadequate when it is most needed. (3) Demands on medical care increase without the financial capacity to deliver the care. In addition, limited numbers of professionals and facilities are available to deliver services, and few health professionals have the ability to work with other systems of service, including the restorative/rehabilitation.

The recovery or comeback phase of illness is handled haphazardly in our health care system, except for its immediate and physically oriented relationship to acute care. Any ill person may not get linked with rehabilitation services. He or she may not get put on the comeback trail because there is not enough money, because there seems to be no real reason to spend money in this way, or because the patient has not been urged or asked to do so by the attending physician. In the United States, getting services is a gambler's game, decided by a throw of fate's dice.

Summary

Comeback, or recovery, phases of illness are not well served if they last longer than a few months, either clinically or in regard to rehabilitation. Rehabilitation services are also restricted in the scope of their mandated coverage of types of disability and disease. Yet even short recoveries from severe acute phases, as well as repeated ones, present many psychological, social, and even clinical difficulties to the ill and their families. Several failures at comebacks can result in additional acute periods or further deterioration.

The first case presented in this chapter highlights the many work arrangements that may have to be made even for a short-term disability, as well as the fragility of such arrangements if the recovery period is prolonged. The second case shows the conditions for getting few or no rehabilitation services and the consequences of this failure for recovery. The third case, about a successful comeback, illustrates ways in which the health care system failed, even in clinical terms.

All of these cases reflect the acute care orientation of physicians and of the health care system in general. Various forms of counseling either do not exist or do not reach recovering patients—certainly not when they are beyond the more or less immediate postacute period of illness. The same is true for financial aid, whether for particular medical services, to counter the loss of a job, or to obtain paid assistance at home. Furthermore, the system is likely to break down even for comeback periods of medium length, with regard to the close or periodic monitoring of physical status that is necessary for a substantial proportion of these ill people. If the system does break down, their recoveries are less successful than they should be, take longer, or put the ill at risk again more quickly and severely.

7

∗ ∗ ∗ ∗ ∗

Holding One's Own

If someone is chronically ill, a stable physiological or physical state is desired. Granted that a given illness is not curable, we hope that at least things won't get worse. "Things" here refers to the illness course, the intrusiveness of symptoms, or disability. After an acute phase, what is aimed for is a swift and durable recovery to whatever level of functioning is now possible. If a person's condition has begun to worsen or is well along in its deterioration, we pray at least for intermittent periods of stability.

From the health professionals' point of view, the acute, recovery, and deteriorating phases are typically the most difficult, for then medical and nursing efforts are required. Once the patient has been properly stabilized, then—unless the condition remains permanently or persistently fragile—one can leave it up to nature, to the regimen, and to the ill themselves. These last phases contain a world of ambiguity, however. In this chapter we attempt to specify and illustrate what it means to leave things up to the ill, their regimen, and nature.

When viewed from the theoretical standpoint outlined in Chapter Five, the maintenance of stability may necessitate very careful management that calls for effective and durable work arrangements. This is not, as we shall see, always possible to ensure.

Moreover, from the perspective of the ill persons, an apt motto for the stable phase might well be: The illness is not (or no longer) in focus, but it is always there in the background affecting how you live your life. An incurable illness becomes conditional, framing and constraining what living and life can be for the ill. The illness becomes conditional in varying degrees, too, for spouses, intimates, and other family members.

The basic issue during stable periods is for the ill to dovetail their stabilizing regimens and disability with the ongoing patterns of their lives. If the regimen is relatively nonintrusive, not taking up too much time or energy or involving the efforts of others, one is very lucky. However, many regimens and disabilities require establishing and maintaining physical and social arrangements. These involve relationships of space, time, work, and persons. Moreover, people who must live with their long-term illnesses somehow must develop routine patterns of managing the major features of their illnesses. Underpinning their routine management patterns, nevertheless, are various arrangements that permit the management work to get done more or less consistently and successfully.

Supporting these routines also is a great amount of accumulated personal knowledge about the uniqueness of one's body and its reactions to specific drugs, types of activities, and environmental conditions like wind, cold, smoke, or the density of a crowded street. The ill also learn how to supplement their prescribed regimens by properly monitoring their bodily cues. These point to immediate or impending trouble. The ill also need to have developed modes of acting for the prevention of bodily deterioration. All of these activities usually become part of people's routines, becoming second nature to them. If people do not act sensitively, sensibly, and to some extent automatically, trouble may lie ahead.

Stability is threatened by occasional dips and drops in physiological condition, and these must be prevented from becoming a genuine crisis. The preventive strategies do not consist simply of medical or nursing interventions but of personally organized actions. These, as well as monitoring bodily signs, involve the cooperation of marital partners, other family members, and even friends and neighbors. This can be seen in the instance of diabetic or hemophiliac children, who must be watched closely by literally everyone: parents, siblings, neighbors, teachers.

A major contributor to stability is a cooperative spouse or other intimate, who may not necessarily be involved in the everyday illness management but shares in its division of labor. These participants also act as agents in a variety of roles, depending on the nature of the illness: controlling agents for careless or tempted diabetics, protection agents for people with severe epilepsy, and so on. For continued stability, other conditions that can be crucial are adequate financing, appropriate housing, an accommodating job, a network of cooperative and sociable friends or kin, and the supportive resources of good counsel (lay or professional) and effective therapy.

For all that, maintaining the equilibrium of a physiological state is precarious even for the most fortunate of the chronically ill. This equilibrium can be upset by various contingencies. Some arise from worsening illness, some from the exigencies of life. Each time the illness becomes more threatening or difficult to manage, the existing routines and arrangements that undergird stability are affected. The same is true when the ill become divorced, are widowed, find it necessary to move to a new city, lose close friends, or see their savings dwindle because of medical expenses.

In light of the foregoing considerations, several questions should be kept in mind while reading the case illustrations that follow.

1. What is the set of arrangements that is keeping the ill and their nonprofessional helpers going?
2. What are the contributory structural and interactional conditions, including use of professional services?
3. If the arrangements are breaking down, or have broken down in the past, why and how?
4. What assistance do they now need, or have they needed, from the health care system? Did they have or are they receiving it? If not, why not?

These questions are designed to bring into sharp focus how and why work and arrangements persist or break down, and what services offered by the American health system contribute to the success or failure of the management work.

The Fitzgeralds: An Explicit
Marital Bargain but a Precarious Balance

When this couple first met at a Quaker fellowship church meeting thirty-one years ago, she found him attractive and musically talented. He found her congenial, creative, and sharing of his artistic interests. Shortly thereafter, he was very helpful to her attempt to found a local recreational program for the handicapped. Although suffering from muscular dystrophy, she could still walk, having begun the slow descent into further disablement only three years before. A decade later, she would start using a cane, then a walker, and finally an electric wheelchair. He had ulcerative colitis and also displayed clear signs of schizophrenia. His family strenuously opposed the marriage because she had become disabled. (She had no parents of her own to convince.) She decided to marry "because he was so committed to what I was committed to. I thought our lives were going in the same direction. I knew jolly well I couldn't do it all by myself. I thought if I could find someone who had the same ideas that I might be able to do it. . . . We both thought our lives were going in the same direction, we both needed support."

Thus, they made what can be fairly termed a bargain. Later they would strike another, a more explicit one. Seven years after the marriage, she began to discover the full implications of that first contract. His ulcerative colitis became so bad that he underwent an ileostomy operation; it was she who had to decide whether he was to be operated on, since "he was too ill [mentally] to decide." Without the operation, she was advised, he would surely die of colitis; if it were performed, he ran a great chance of suffering a mental breakdown. "There was a whole panel of doctors telling me those things." Shortly after the operation, he had such a bad breakdown that his psychiatrist committed him to a mental hospital. Soon after, the psychiatrist flatly counseled her to get a divorce, since her husband would never recover sufficiently to return to her. She got a divorce.

Thereafter she knit her life together slowly. Three years after the divorce, her former husband's psychiatrist appeared, literally, on her doorstep.

He said, "Well, David is doing better and we think
it is your duty to let him come home." I said,
"What! You just told me three years ago to forget
it. I have my own life now." I said I had made other
arrangements. Well, he said, "I want you to think
it over." Well, I was really having a hard time
[then]. So I said I will think it over. I had ten ses-
sions with him. Then I agreed that I would let
David come home on one condition.

That one condition had two parts: he would stay under psychiatric treatment, and there would be a clear financial arrangement. "I spelled it all out . . . that what was mine was mine.
He could [eventually] have his Social Security. His family as-
sured me that they would give us some money to live on." When
his father died a few years later, her husband came into a trust
which gave him monthly payments. He went back to work then
and continued for ten years. She was no longer working, and
had never built up any Social Security savings. She concluded,
"In the end, I guess I am grateful to the psychiatrist because
I really couldn't make it on my own. Over the long haul, I
wouldn't have been able to. I was doing it then but I was having a hard time, financially and everything."

They have been able to afford his psychiatric treatments
as well as her occasional visits to a psychologist. They can also
afford a housekeeper-attendant five days a week. The attendant
also bathes her and helps her on and off the toilet. When her
husband helps to move her, sometimes "he is pretty rough on
me," so rough that occasionally her body gets bruised. "Sometimes he gets so spaced out so he seems like a piece of furniture.
It's kind of tough having to depend on someone who is just not
there." However, her complaints about the physical aspects of
their relationship are minimal.

Her husband also bathes her on Sundays, helps her in
and out of the auto, drives, takes her by wheelchair up short
flights of stairs when necessary, helps her in the bathroom, does
the shopping and household errands, and does the gardening.
When he is working in the garden, she can signal to him if she

needs him by pressing a buzzer. He also does the family's accounting and pays the bills, because she doesn't like to, whereas he enjoys those tasks. However, she worries a bit because "sometimes he pays a bill three times, sometimes he doesn't pay at all. I am not sure he can handle it but so far nobody has complained, and he has to have something to do. I am not good at it, I don't like it." She does keep a sharp eye on the Blue Cross bill, knowing how disastrous it would be if they lost their health insurance.

Her part in the marital division of labor is considerably more difficult than his. Besides doing the general overseeing of the household and preparing the shopping lists, she does things especially for him. First of all, she closely monitors whether he is taking his medications on schedule and makes him do so when he does not. She insists he stay off alcohol because of his drugs. (She threatens him by saying, "I am going to tell your psychiatrist." As she says, "I have to have leverage somehow. . . . I use what works." Her own psychologist has counseled this tough stance.) She also protects him against stress, especially financial, by helping to find solutions to problems. When he gets extremely restless, "I insist he take some medication. Then I find out what is causing it. Usually it has to do with money. . . . Then I try to get rid of the cause." She also needs, in her own interest, to keep him in very good health. Understanding this issue perfectly well, he agrees not to climb ladders. He knows too that, if possible, he shouldn't pass along any of his colds, since they could be extremely dangerous and even life-threatening for her.

From time to time, her monitoring and managing of him bring into the marital drama both his psychiatrist and her psychologist, and even their friends. For instance, one summer he read a book called *The Intimate Enemy*, "and he got this idea that if you are going to really relate to each other you have to fight a lot. So he started fighting all the time." A friend suggested that his medications might be causing this argumentativeness and advised her to ask his psychiatrist to change the medications (which he did). She also visited her psychologist for counseling on how to get him off his "intimate enemy" idea.

Sometimes he goes off on tangents that would cost precious money—recently, for example, he wished to take up what she considers an utterly foolish diet that would cost seven hundred dollars. She resisted his plan firmly. For support, she called on an ally whom she had occasionally relied on before: the trustee of his fund. On this kind of financial issue, she says, "I am not all by myself."

This incident suggests some of the price she pays in keeping her part of the marital bargain. There is in fact a long list of particulars that she did not foresee. "I have to tell him what to do all the time, he is not very self-directed." Every day she makes out a shopping list. "It is to keep him busy, because if he is not busy he gets wild." She helps him "sort out his priorities, what he should do, ought not to do . . . that he keeps his appointments. . . . I have to watch all the time. . . . I have to take all the responsibility." For instance, she has to remind him to get gas for the car, to walk the dog, to feed the cat. "It is a great weight sometimes. It is like having a kid. He won't take responsibility for anything."

She sometimes grows weary of all the strain of planning and monitoring his care; she grows angry, too. "I just blow my stack. I am not always kind about it, and that makes me feel guilty." She took a course in "assertiveness," and found that for a while it made her feel less guilty. On days when he is a bit depressed, she rather likes this because this gives her some relief from pressure, and she can "get things done. . . . To tell the truth I like it." A few months before, when her husband was constantly hyperactive, she became dizzy from tension. Her therapist hazarded that she had been holding her breath because of tension, and suggested she try deep breathing; the symptoms have since disappeared. The main problem for her is "the uncertainty of the whole thing. When he is in one of those moods, I don't know what he is going to do. He is very careless. He could burn the house down. He might hurt himself or me, or get the neighbors mad at him. It is just the total unpredictability."

He knows perfectly well how his mental disabilities affect her, and he feels contrite and guilty about this. He also knows and appreciates how dependent he is on her: "She sustains me. I feed off of her. . . . I think I have emotionally leached her because of my needs and my trying to solve my problems has made things worse for her. . . . I am unhappy about that. Being unhappy means that I am a problem." However, he faults her for his being unable to share his inner life and problems with her. "That's just not possible. She's a cheerful person who likes to be happy and does not want to talk" about their respective disabilities. As he says, "mine is an inner struggle primarily." He finds he cannot talk to her about this, for it depresses her. But he understands and has empathy for her, reasoning that "my natural struggle for my own independence has killed us off. I feel that sincerely. I don't know what to do about it. My inner struggle, I am not going to give up." Instead of talking about this with her, he talks with his psychiatrist. His wife disappoints him in yet another way that is related to his feeling of having leached her. She has somehow lost much of the creativity that he so admired at the very outset of their relationship, thirty years ago. Her life is not so active any more, she spends more time watching TV, and so on.

Despite the difficulties of their relationship, and with themselves in relation to it, each finds it is not at all a bad life that they live. They share activities together. They have many good friends. They are helpful to each other. Furthermore, they are honest enough to say to themselves (and to the interviewer) that their mutual bargain is a fair one. Thus, he says, "I think we have a pretty good life. I am not unhappy about it." Her feelings are perhaps more complex. When she talks to a friend who is also having a difficult marriage, "I tell her to look at it as a job, a well-paying job. Indeed, that is how I view our situation, and I'm darn glad to get it. . . . He is affectionate. There is nothing there behind it. But the gesture is there and I am glad to get it." They also have "a real sense of community" with their shared friends, "and that really helps." They are "not truly together, but we are together in our activities." Whenever she gets terribly frustrated and angry, "I look on the other side and say, would I like to be by myself on welfare with the Reagan cuts? So when you look at the alternatives. Besides, I have no

family. I have no place to go. I have no place to go. This way
I have somebody that needs me. (I never had any brothers or
sisters. My parents died.) Otherwise what is the point.''

And so they are both locked into a modus vivendi built
on a voluntary exchange of help and obligation rather than on
deep affection. What are their expectations about this relationship? The answer is that they expect it to continue exactly as
is until one of them dies. They both expect that her death will
precede his; at the age of sixty-one, she has, they estimate,
perhaps five or six years remaining, based on what they know
about life probabilities for people with muscular dystrophy. However, he worries about what would happen to her financially
if he died first. ''At least half of our income will disappear from
her use.'' She would have the house and what belongs to him,
but his trust, he believes, would revert to his brothers and sisters.
It is their plan to live as comfortably as possible, not stinting,
until her death. ''That is our agreement. We have decided on
that. This house is beyond our means. We are living here on
our capital, phasing it out gradually so that it is zero when she
dies. Then our plan is that I go find a job.'' His projection for
himself thereafter involves joining a cooperative live-together
group, earning his board and keep by doing some gardening.

Her version of this plan—essentially another contract—
is as follows. After she had fallen ill a couple of times, the trustee
of his trust was worried ''because there was no plan, so we finally
got his niece to help him work out a plan.'' But ''there is no
plan if he goes first. Nobody seems to be worried about that
but me. I don't think about it too much. I would hope the family
would let the trust continue until I die, but they might decide
not to give me anything. I know I would get the house. Outside of that I don't know.'' However, ''I don't think much about
it because the odds are that I will go first, because I have had
close calls the last three months. Not that I am looking forward
to dying but people with muscular dystrophy don't live much
over sixty.'' If she does not die first, she simply assumes that
she would go on welfare. Both were on welfare during the early
years of their marriage, before they were rescued by the allowance from his father and later by the trust payments.

Commentary

Following the series of questions listed at the beginning of this chapter, let us address the general issue of what this oddly matched couple's common enterprise implies for a programmatic health policy that would be applicable to the chronically ill.

Arrangements. Several arrangements support the current stability of the couple's respective illnesses, as well as the management itself. First, a firm contract stipulates that (a) he will be under continuous psychiatric care, and (b) there will be a clear financial arrangement between them, with some allowance of money coming regularly from his father. Such an explicit contract shows that both parties are aware of the basis of their marital relationship and what it may take to sustain it. Several years of marriage before their divorce showed her the more specific details of what would make a remarriage workable.

A second arrangement that evolved between them involves the everyday housework and the chronic illness management. He is responsible for manual tasks, she for mental ones. She does the mental work for him and acts as a controlling and monitoring agent for his mental illness; he does the physical work of aiding and easing her bodily movements as well as some of the everyday household chores. His tasks include helping her move from one place to another, bathing her once a week, shopping, doing household errands, and doing the gardening. Her tasks include preparing the shopping lists, monitoring his taking of medications, keeping him off alcohol, protecting him against psychological stress, keeping him from doing foolish things, helping him sort out priorities, and keeping track of his appointments. It is important to understand that this set of working arrangements is essential to the management of their respective illnesses, keeping each relatively stable, and that the everyday living aspects of the arrangements are a necessary condition for the illness management.

Their third arrangement is the agreement to "live to the hilt" on their income, come what may, rather than cutting back on expenses. This enables him to visit a psychiatrist regularly—a necessity for keeping his condition stable and undoubtedly also for keeping their marriage together. The money also allows her to receive psychological therapy—apparently also a necessity for her to carry on in the face of the considerable strain of living with someone who has to be monitored so closely. Without the extra financing, this couple would not be able to afford the housekeeper-attendant for her. This would create much more work for him to do, which would become increasingly stressful for him and eventually for their marital relationship. The medical insurance that their income pays for eases their anxieties about what might happen if either became temporarily ill. It also helps to pay the medical bills for professional services that help to keep her condition relatively stable.

Structural and Interactional Conditions. The chief contributory condition is the financial arrangement of the lifetime monthly allowance and trust money from his father. Among their resources, also, are their therapists' services, without which the marriage would soon collapse. They themselves constitute the chief resources for managing each other's illness, for neither the money nor the therapists would be sufficient to keep this marriage functioning or their illnesses under control. A great deal of illness-related work and intrafamily agreements are required. Her alert attention to him keeps his mental condition from worsening. She acts as a control agent by buffering him against stress, monitoring adherence to his regimen, and giving him tasks to keep him occupied. Sometimes, when there is a contest for control between them, she calls on outside control agents for backup, including even the trustee official. She also safeguards his physical health. In doing so she helps to maintain her own, since a severe respiratory infection or a bout of flu could place her life in jeopardy.

Without her, he would sooner or later end up in a mental institution. But without him, she might not be able to live alone, unless she had enough income to hire a full-time, physically strong housekeeper or attendant. Her husband knows this, understands their bargain, and cooperates with both her monitoring of his regimen and her efforts to keep his psyche as stable as possible. She puts up with a good deal in order to keep up her end of the bargain, and to get whatever satisfaction she can out of their relationship. He perhaps has less to put up with, but he is committed in much the same way. Their mutual commitment and their acting as essential resources for one another are partly a pragmatic and partly a somewhat sentimental matter. Understandably, the pragmatic attitude takes precedence. Its results are probably so effective just because they expect so little from each other in the way of intense communication and deep intimacy. They have much invested in this relationship, and allowing it to die might well mean a kind of foreclosing on life for each.

This minimal but genuine sentimental attachment has been buttressed by an important factor outside the more positive internal workings of their relationship. This is their talent for establishing and maintaining a network of friends. This appears to have been necessary for reducing tensions engendered by their living and working together. Over the years, their close friends, especially hers, have offered occasional helpful counsel, sometimes at critical junctures.

Breakdown of Arrangements. Because of the strong cementing force of their symbiotic relations, their respective illnesses are relatively stable. Yet both aspects of the total relationship are actually in precarious balance. To begin with, the great weakness of the symbiosis—of their functioning as a work team— is that it rests on their ability to do their jobs adequately. This in turn depends largely on their respective illness conditions. A drastic deterioration in either person's condition could threaten their working relationship. For instance, if he were to suffer an acute breakdown that led to a brief hospitalization, she would need a temporary substitute for his manpower. If he were to have a more severe or total breakdown, she would be in deep trouble, as she was many years ago, after they divorced because of his breakdown. She would then need a permanent replacement for him. The services of a full-time attendant could be purchased with money from their small savings or from the monthly trust payments. However, if he actually died, though she would be permitted to continue living in the house, she would

literally have no income. Her only recourse would be to go on
Medicaid and enter a nursing home. It is only her husband's
life and stable condition that keep her from such a fate.

Consider, however, what would happen if his condition
remained stable but her own deteriorated greatly. She would
have less energy and probably less alertness, and so face increasing difficulty in monitoring his regimen and controlling his mental state and physical health. His condition would probably
worsen until it affected his physical handling of her and his social
interaction with her. In turn, this would worsen her physical
condition and her ability to monitor and control him. Under
these conditions, they could well move into a catastrophic spiral.

Their symbiotic relationship depends also on keeping the
tension between them at a minimum. This is achieved, as we
have seen, through much control on her part, the efforts of two
therapists, and support from their friends. It is also achieved
because of their clear awareness of the necessity for their mutual
bargain, and because of their minimal demands on each other
aside from the basic elements of that bargain. Their ability to
levy the agreed-on demands on each other depends on the stability of their respective illness conditions. The simultaneous stability of their marital relations and their illnesses seems to be in
delicate equilibrium and its future extremely uncertain.

Assistance. What kind of assistance have they needed from
the health care system? Have they received it? If not, why not?
These questions will be approached first from the practitioner's
point of view, and then from the policymaker's.

A range of physicians and therapists, the mental hospital,
and medical insurance, at a price, are available to this couple.
Yet what additional assistance will they need if she either deter-
iorates or dies? What if she lives longer than they expect and
their funding is insufficient to cover therapists, housekeeper,
or attendant? Currently, they could well use sensitive family
counseling that would carefully avoid disturbing their bargain
and not insist on greater marital intimacy. Such counseling
might reduce his rough physical handling of her when he is trying to help with her physical care. Yet the advice they really

need most urgently is that of a counselor who thinks in trajectory terms. The trajectory of neither partner is likely to remain stable once hers starts to go downhill. Thinking ahead to the options that lie before them is not easy for either partner. Yet realism is called for. What can they think of or do right now that might forestall the most difficult episodes and avoid the most catastrophic consequences?

It is important for any counselor to understand that the great strength of their relationship lies in its division of labor. If that division becomes too unbalanced, too asymmetrical, their marital arrangements could explode.

In the long run, professional aid in keeping them together as a working team would need to begin soon, continue periodically, and increase when the trajectory of either begins to threaten marital havoc. The precise content of the counsel offered them should, of course, depend on the trajectory phase not only of the illness but of the work and worker relationships involved in managing the illness. Unfortunately, neither spouse recognizes—probably having never been advised—that such professional counseling services are available to them and are probably needed. Middle-class friends and medically oriented physicians apparently have not recognized this either.

We turn now to the broader policy issues raised by this couple's story. By and large, the American health care system entered supportively in the form of the psychiatrist and her medical care, as well as their medical insurance. This is offset, however, by the weakness of their overall situation, which is hardly helped by the current operation of our health care system. Indeed, their weakness reflects some of the system's weaknesses. While they have a middle-class income, right now they are playing a gambler's game, living to the edge of their income and assuming that she has only a few years to live. If their money runs out, they will need to sell their house, and perhaps eventually to go on welfare, unless they are rescued financially by his father's estate. In four years she will be eligible for Medicare, but this will not be adequate if she becomes debilitated or if he develops an illness that affects his ability to help with her physical care. Even if they can maintain their health insurance, it will hardly pay for the bodily aid that she needs. Also, as middle-class people, they will not know their way around the agency maze; nor, despite their education, will either be in the proper physical or mental condition to gather the requisite information that might ease their path through the maze. It is not likely either that their friends will know more about this, but their friends might have more energy to help to figure out the system. They are very lucky to have the money to pay for health insurance, especially if deterioration begins before they reach sixty-five. But if their money had lasted only until their mid fifties, what then?

If he suffers a severe or permanent mental breakdown, dies first, or even leaves her, she will become one of the single elderly sick—the status enjoyed by the majority of chronically ill women. What does our health system offer to those people, especially when they have little or no money? This question pertains not merely to the adequate financing of medical care but to the availability of a much larger range of services. These include rehabilitation services, such as she needs even now, a driver to take her to and from medical facilities, and various housekeeping services. Right now her husband provides unpaid labor—the usual role of the spouse—thus saving government considerable expense. When the healthy or healthier spouse dies, then the widow or widower is up against the wall, given the contingencies of American family life and the character of our health care system.

Ironically, in the United States, state governments provide at least a modicum of long-term care for the mentally ill. So, if the husband were to have a severe mental collapse, he would end up in a state mental hospital or, if it were less severe, in a community facility. If she dies first, he will surely need community mental health services at least. If he dies first, the American health care system offers her only welfare status and custodial care in an institution.

This couple's socioeconomic status is clearly middle-class, even if they have little or no savings and no earnings because of their disabilities. Though they are not destitute and their illnesses are not unstable, their story points to some of the consequences of living in a country that provides relatively little for people like them if they become destitute or their illnesses become unstable—or if, as intimated above, they become single persons through divorce or death.

The Smiths: The End of Long-Term Stability

For middle- or low-income couples and families, our health system can ultimately become very cruel. There is a tendency to assume that relative financial security and the presence of a spouse together mitigate the severity of the chronically ill person's social and economic situation. The failures of the nation's health system, however, leave the chronically ill open to a destructive fate. Their marital and family relationships can be profoundly affected by the illness and its management. For the ill and their families, three fates become grave possibilities. The first is that they become impoverished and go on welfare, either because they have exhausted their savings or because going on welfare is a prerequisite for placing the ill person in a nursing home. A second possibility is that they will have to settle for a greatly lowered standard of living, a much impaired quality of life, and even—through the dwindling or destruction of their savings—the collapse of their dreams and plans for the future. A third possibility is the dissolution of the marriage.

A striking example of the last possibility is the situation of a couple that lived happily together for over two decades until the wife could no longer bear the physical and psychological burdens of his care. The husband had suffered a catastrophic accident and become a quadriplegic shortly after their marriage. Because he was in the army, he received all the benefits of his service, including excellent and lifelong Veterans Administration (VA) medical-nursing care. Even the early psychological and sexual counseling seemed very useful to the couple. From the outset of his disability and its associated illnesses, she did much of his physical care, for he could do little of it. This care included helping him in his defecation and clean-up routines, getting him in and out of bed, dressing and bathing him, nursing him when he was sick, and helping him in and out of his wheelchair and maneuvering it whenever they left the house. In the first weeks after his accident, the VA hospital staff taught her some aspects of his care and daily management; nevertheless, she was really very much on her own in learning how to do these things. All of them she did with great care and commitment, for the couple was very much in love until his death.

She had no backstop in her physical labor, no real assistance. They tried paid attendants but decided fairly quickly that they much preferred that she do the work. There were three reasons for their decision. An attendant meant a massive invasion of their privacy, especially acute in their case: they had established a cocoon-like existence together, based on intimacy and shared work. Moreover, they discovered that none of the attendants whom they had hired was sufficiently sensitive or skilled in handling his severe physical conditions. Finally, there did not seem to be enough money from disability payments or his pension to warrant the extra expenditure. This threw virtually all the physical burden on her. They had no kin living nearby, nor anyone who could cover for her when she needed relief. Ironically, her chief respite came when he was hospitalized during occasional medical emergencies. Thus she had no one to help when she had the flu, no one to spell her at night so that she could get a restful sleep, no one to take over at home even temporarily when the shopping had to be done. Her difficulties were compounded by a lack of nonworking women friends. In any event, this couple was so busy at home that they had no time or energy, nor the mobility, to build the usual circle of supportive friends.

Twenty-three years after their wedding, it took much more labor to keep his condition stable. At the same time, this forty-five-year-old woman, now undergoing menopause, no longer had the unbounded energy of her youth. She also developed a severe allergic skin reaction that kept her indoors during the summer. When her husband had another emergency that took him back into the hospital, "I kind of quit. . . . It really did burn me out. . . . It was just too much pressure." Her allergic reaction made her confront his dependence on her health: "The hospital wouldn't take him in because *I* got sick. . . . I was losing confidence that I could keep this all together.'' Each new emergency frightened her more. Finally she said to herself, "I can't take any more." She placed him in a long-term VA unit, where he died some months later. Her own financial security was not threatened because his pension would sustain her.

Shortly before she gave up the struggle, the couple had tried to get assistance from various agencies. As she described it:

> We tried quite a few things. I was trying for help during these last five years. We looked into a home health aide. I took a five-hour class one day a week, and what a rigmarole to get everyone to overlap so that I could get coverage during that time. Because of insurance problems, the nurse couldn't do health aide work, she couldn't wash him. A health aide couldn't feed him or give him his medications. So I had to have a nurse come and I could get the one feeding in that morning. It really threw the whole day off for his feedings. I had to squish them in the rest of the day. The health aide could wash him and dress him but couldn't get him up. I would come home and find him in bed and had to get him up and feed him right away. We had to overlap the time the therapist came. And trying to keep them all busy—it was such a rigmarole to get one person to do enough to make it worthwhile. They had to come for so many hours and there was only so much you could do squished together that was a help. We just forgot the whole thing. Then we did use the health aide program this summer when I was feeling kind of down. But they had allowed it for so long and then they would no longer provide the finances for it. We had meantime changed a lot of ideas of how we would adapt ourselves to it. Then they wouldn't pay for it. I couldn't believe what they charge for those services. Something like thirty dollars an hour.

Even if she had managed to get some relief through such services, it probably would have been far too late to save this marriage.

As he became sicker, her own health and energies broke down. She became increasingly anxious and frightened by his medical emergencies. She had reached the end of her tether. Worst of all was the dissolution of a loving marital relationship. Both spouses were devastated by the parting and by the need to give up and put him in a nursing home. That their situation is not unusual is suggested by the situation of another couple whom we interviewed. The husband had recently become paraplegic and his young wife was embarking on the same fateful journey. She was taking up the wife-attendant role with devotion, commitment, and energy. How long will the marriage last, and with what quality of life? She does not realize that with increasing age, energy diminishes and the ability to do the unending labor decreases.

Another couple reflects the same unfortunate effects of a crippling chronic disability with associated illnesses combined with a strikingly inadequate health care system. This couple's relationship is the opposite of that of the "cocooned" couple, however. Because the husband is very anxious about the daily management of his bodily needs, which are many and need very careful handling, he tends to supervise and to be critical of his wife's skills. This has resulted gradually in increased mutual irritability, tension, conflict, and psychological distance, so that she feels more of an attendant than a wife. It is perhaps only their children who keep this marriage going. A very difficult health situation is combined with a health care system that not only has failed to reach them with services but is not prepared to act effectively even if it could have offered very useful services.

Sometimes these couples are given good counsel. Yet if the resources for carrying out the advice are lacking, their burdens will not be eased. There is an institutional vacuum— available services do not meet what the ill and their intimates actually need to lighten their burdens and give them a better quality of life. The experiences that we have described occur over and over again. Yet the health services are not there to be delivered. These cases show clearly that our health care system is predominantly—almost completely—focused on servicing acute care. This it certainly does well, at least for some populations. It does not at all, however, confront the problem of maintaining stability of illness conditions.

Summary

In this chapter, we have seen that keeping a severe chronic illness stabilized is not a simple matter, nor is it necessarily accomplished merely by putting "the patient" on a proper regimen. The basic issue for the ill during their stable phases is to dovetail their stabilizing regimens and disability with the ongoing patterns of their lives. Many regimens and disabilities require establishing and maintaining physical and social arrangements. These involve relationships of space, time, persons, work, and of course routines or standard ways of carrying out regimens, monitoring symptoms, and maintaining life. A major contribution to stabilization is a cooperative spouse or other intimate or caretaker. Other contributing conditions are adequate financing, appropriate housing, an accommodating employer and work colleagues, good counseling services, and effective therapy.

Two cases have illustrated the issues of maintaining stability when one or both marital partners have a severe chronic illness. The first case portrays an oddly matched couple (one is a schizophrenic and the other has muscular dystrophy) who live in precarious stability—as individuals and as a marital pair. The case brings out the sustaining arrangements that make their respective and mutual stability possible, as well as the great dangers to stability. For this couple, potential as well as actual weaknesses in the health care system are evident. The second case illustrates the end-of-the-road plight of a long-stabilized couple. This case is typical of a large number of the elderly ill. These people gradually experience a decrease of their resources, including finances, energy, and helping friends. The conditions sustaining any continued stability become weaker and weaker, and unstable periods become more frequent and momentous. Ultimately, these people are likely to face impoverishment. The health care system as presently constituted fails in important ways to answer their needs. Indeed, it does not reach them with much beyond strictly medical types of care.

The stable phases of severe chronic illness trajectories are precarious. They are sustained not only by physiological condition but by unremitting care. An acute care perspective almost totally misses the necessity for supportive services during these periods.

8

$\ast \ast \ast \ast \ast$

Coping with
Periods of Instability

Another trajectory phase is the unstable phase. It is a trajectory phase because it involves not only a person's physiology but also his or her work. We call this phase *unstable* to distinguish it from more or less stable conditions, as well as from periods of acute illness when people are in medical crises or emergencies.

Some illnesses typically fluctuate, either in terms of intrusiveness of symptoms or in a deeper physical sense. This fluctuation may occur periodically, even daily. Severe arthritis is an example of a condition that typically evidences frequent ups and downs. People suffering from racking migraines or recurrent, severe back pain also usually seem to experience periods when they are stable and others when their symptoms come and go in intensity. In severe allergies or asthma, periods of stability alternate with periods of considerable instability. The latter are often baffling, maddeningly intrusive on life, and even life-threatening if they are not properly managed—or if the body itself does not somehow mysteriously manage to pull itself together. Some people are subject to two or more chronic illnesses simultaneously. If one is stable while the other is unstable, the unstable illness may affect the stable condition, resulting in a spiral of destabilization.

These periods are causally linked with changes in physiological condition, of course, but various behavioral and social

99

conditions also contribute to those changes. Carelessly kept regimens, poor monitoring, inadequate illness management, and inappropriate environmental settings can all contribute to instability. Calculating one's physical capacities or putting or finding oneself in a difficult social situation can also exacerbate symptoms or further damage a physical condition. Since these unstable periods have great and even momentous consequences for behavior, mood, and identity, they should not be conceived of in terms of acute care nor wholly as a matter of medical management.

Yet it is useful to analyze briefly the difference between acute and unstable phases. During the former, health professionals tend to be the major agents for managing an illness. Meanwhile, disturbances in the ill person's life, and in that of the spouse, have a fair chance of being mitigated by the cooperation of family members, friends, neighbors, and even fellow employees and employers. The latter may allow periods of sick leave, and colleagues may willingly take up slack in the work. If the disruption in the ill person's life requires changes in the division of labor between spouses or within the family, this can usually be more or less accomplished by shifting tasks around. Relatives will help with the children, friends with the shopping, and so on. Of course, expectations about the activities or work of the ill themselves are suspended: they are "sick" and cannot be expected to carry on normal work, jobs, or even perhaps their usual mental activities.

Picture now someone who has entered an unstable period. If this is the first of such phases, the work and behavior of others may not be very different from a typical acute phase of illness. But if the instability continues, what then? Cooperative support tends to dwindle; after all, others have their own lives to live. Furthermore, if the instability is succeeded by a period of stability—with the reinstitution of normal family, job, and social relations—but new periods of disruption occur, what will be the result? Not only are friends, associates, and even family members less cooperative, they may also be less understanding, less inclined to give credence to the fact that the person is really sick— or at least that sick. Physicians also, unless they believe there are genuine indicators of destabilization, are likely to discount complaints, or explain away slightly worsened symptoms as having a psychosomatic origin. As for employers and fellow workers, whether they are understanding or not, their patience cannot override the exigencies of the work situation. Repeated sick leaves without pay may be granted, but no salary will flow in. If the sickness occurs frequently, the ill are likely to drag themselves to work anyway, which sets the stage for further physical destabilization.

Meanwhile, they are likely to resort to routines that they have found to help, or believe may help, mitigate the manifestations of illness or at least shorten the period of destabilization. Sometimes, of course, the routines work, but sometimes they do not. How long does one endure instability before deciding that the routines are not working? If they do not work, the ill ask themselves, "What can I do now?" They may request that their physicians change their medications or regimens, or ask friends and acquaintances who have similar illnesses what they themselves do.

Moreover, while life is coming increasingly to a standstill (as we shall describe below), the ill may well be becoming worn out both physically and psychologically. Worst yet, they may believe their basic illness conditions are actually deteriorating, perhaps permanently. Desperate for relief of symptoms, and for relief from their anxiety or panic, they typically turn to other physicians or to practitioners who offer alternative forms of care. It should be no surprise that shopping around is characteristic of people who suffer from arthritis, rheumatism, severe allergies, or "back problems." Bizarre alternative treatments may be tried: "Who knows—the physicians certainly don't!" At this stage of medical and psychological stress, the ill are very vulnerable to far-out medical ideologies, some harmful, some costly as well as useless. Some alternative treatments require the ill to adapt their life-styles, changing to a drastically different diet or substantially remodeling a house to control hitherto uncontrollable allergies. If these methods are judged to work— that is, if one's physical condition is restabilized—there may still be a question in others' minds as to whether there really was any causal connection between the new treatments or altered life-style and the physical improvement. This skepticism may persist even if the stable period lasts for a long time. Moreover, if the ill suffer from more than one illness, they themselves almost inevitably have the responsibility for managing several medical regimens that they may suspect are actually interfering with or undercutting one another. They may also worry about the possible side effects—including a long-term accumulation of drug effects.

Meanwhile, what about their everyday lives? The usual scenario is that household chores and duties are put off or partly neglected until later; socializing is curtailed; immediate plans are abandoned or deferred. Later, unless the destabilized periods are very frequent, the ill will catch up with everything. After a period of catching up, everything more or less goes back to normal. Spouses or other intimates may need to be extremely flexible in their adaptation to the fluctuations or temporary alterations of unstable physical and social conditions. They may have to go along with the supposition that a changed life-style is the only alternative for their partner. If both persons suffer from chronic illnesses, this is likely to affect greatly how successfully things can be worked out either temporarily or permanently. All in all, the new arrangements made by the ill, with the cooperation of spouses or paid services of other people, are ultimately short-lived and fragile, vulnerable to a host of destructive contingencies. The term *instability* includes the instability of the arrangements that frequently are what really permit these ill people to carry on.

Jan and Tom: Long-Term Instability

Jan and Tom have been married for two years, since their late twenties. She is a writer and part-time college teacher, and he is a freelance consultant who does most of his work at home. Jan has suffered for fifteen years from migraine headaches. Until recently their cause was unknown, but now they are believed to result from an immune deficiency disease. From time to time she has symptoms of headache, wild, unprovoked anger, personality distortion, "spaciness," and disorientation.

For eleven years, her headaches were controlled with a form of ergot, to which she had an extreme chemical sensitivity. This drug, along with certain foods, unpurified water, and polluted air, eventually caused a toxic overload that her body, because of the immune deficiency, could not handle. She was getting sicker and sicker.

Two years ago, Jan's physician changed her medical regimen, prescribing smaller, daily prophylactic doses of her drug. This regimen compounded her symptoms. "I thought I was mentally ill and so did Tom. I was paranoid, really hostile, weepy, volatile, had impulses to dance on table tops and at meetings. I had self-destructive and bizarre impulses." Realizing that something was wrong, she renegotiated her medication dosage, though the physician agreed only reluctantly.

The new regimen seemed to work for about a year. Eventually, however, her behavioral symptoms became so bad that she had to taper off the drug. This apparently brought about a severe headache; the pain was so intense that she wanted to die. However, after three months, she was completely off drugs, and felt "terrific." She even lost some weight. Yet she did not yet feel ready to return to writing. She kept busy doing things around the house.

Eventually, Jan was able to return to her teaching position. Soon, however, she began to get severe headaches again and to feel "sicker and sicker." Although she did not wish to resume taking drugs, she decided to do so because "I was going crazy from the pain." Her bizarre behavior returned. Her neurologist prescribed yet another drug, which seemed to control the headaches and decrease her behavioral manifestations, but only for about three months. At least she was able to return to teaching and writing. Gradually, however, her psychotic-like behavior returned; she thought, "Perhaps it is not the drugs, but I am really nuts." She began to get belligerent at faculty meetings and abrasive with students, as well as feeling physically sick. About this time, she and her husband went away for the weekend. What was supposed to be a great romantic vacation turned out to be a disaster. "I was complaining nonstop about everything. I didn't know where this new personality had emerged from and I didn't like it much. Tom certainly didn't."

Jan returned to her doctor, who told her to stop taking drugs. Once again she had severe headaches, which continued on and off for two months. She was treated with morphine injections and oxygen. During this time, "I was too sick to be left alone in the house because I would throw up so violently that I could pass out and hit my head falling down. I couldn't get anything done in my life and I was desperately clutchy and fearful."

Tom, who had been doing research on Jan's illness, suggested she might have food allergies. Not knowing where to turn, she read a book he had given her about this topic. Because she thought she saw a relationship between what the book said and her symptoms, she went to see an allergist—whom Tom had been urging her to see. The physician agreed that her symptoms pointed to immune deficiency. It was decided that she should be hospitalized for diagnostic testing. She said of this time: "At this point I was ready to check out. I had been through two periods of the status migranosis form of the disease. I sat down with Tom and said, 'I am seriously considering checking out. I promise I won't just leave a suicide note and do it. I promise we will sit down and talk it out. It will be a rational decision. I cannot continue to live this way. I do not have a meaningful life, I do not have work, I am not going to wind up with any friends. It is a serious question to me why you are hanging around. I am not much fun to be with.' I figured I had not tried everything yet and I thought going to the hospital and having the testing would give me some breathing space while I figured out what the hell I wanted to do."

At the hospital, Jan was diagnosed with immune deficiency, as well as several severe allergies. As a result, she and her husband decided to have their house completely remodeled to cut down on dust, pollen, mold, and so on. They also spent considerable money on an extended visit by her to a detoxification center in another state, where she was also put on a drastically altered diet to which she still adheres.

The husband's part in helping to keep her as stable as possible and to get her through the periods of instability was complex and essential. He was primarily responsible for finally getting an accurate set of diagnoses. He also monitored her physical and mental conditions closely for signs that she was moving into one of her periods of destabilization. This is perhaps the principal arrangement that kept their marriage going. If the marriage dissolved, how would Jan manage to live all alone? As Tom said, "Probably the key role that I have played through all of this is a kind of monitoring in terms of the psychological stuff. Is she acting crazy? And if she is, is it because she is reacting against something in the world, is it the drug, or is it some sort of physiological condition? If it is one of these, then I am in some sort of position to try and calm her down." Sometimes, when he could not decide whether the manifestations were mental or physiological, he was thrown into a stressful moral dilemma. "There is a heavy moral responsibility about a thing when one person has to judge the psychological status of another, at any given time, especially when it is a fluctuating entity. I don't know if I am making the right decision. For instance, I don't know if she is just really pissed off at me about something and I say, 'You are nuts at the moment.' I have to be sure of myself, that I am not taking advantage of where she is at. I try to be real careful about that." Another agreement that this couple made was that in public, he would both monitor her mental aberrations and cover for her in interactions, if possible. Nevertheless, she alienated many of their friends with her aggressively critical behavior. In the end, the marriage did not survive the stress of Jan's illness.

As this case illustrates, the hallmark of a very unstable trajectory phase is that life is in disarray, not merely physiologically but socially and biographically. Until this phase has either been conquered or run its clinical course, one has to endure. Under such circumstances, there is plenty of experiential drama. The next case presentation reflects this same drama. However, because this person lives alone, her situation highlights the failings of our health care system for people who are living through intensely unstable periods of illness.

Sue: Sudden and Prolonged Instability

Sue is unmarried and in her mid thirties. She is working toward a doctoral degree in an urban university 2,000 miles away from her family. In the autumn of 1982, she came down with flu that persisted until she was diagnosed at the student health clinic as having an allergy. She had trouble breathing and "ran downhill." Then she had an acute asthma attack. "Before then I thought of myself as a healthy person." Not getting any real relief, she soon left the clinic, transferring to a private physician who did tests for her allergies. By Christmas, she sometimes felt "out of control . . . in outer space." Over the next two years, she suffered many dips, drops, and actual medical crises from her asthma, as well as from osteoporosis and difficulties with menopause, both of which were probably precipitated by her asthma medications.

She now had to manage several illnesses with their involved body systems, symptoms, interventions, and potential side effects. She needed to monitor closely all of these illnesses and the effects of their respective regimens, since the several physicians who treated her did not coordinate her regimens. Moreover, they frequently changed the regimens because they were not working effectively or had untoward side effects. The responsibility for juggling all this management and making decisions about it—except for the actual decisions about regimens—lay completely with her. She had great difficulty in making accurate assessments. Things would get out of control: they seemed to be getting worse, but what was really happening? Which illness was involved? What should she do? Which physician's services should she request? Potential crises occasionally threatened; their management consisted largely in waiting out the episode—just enduring, "hanging in there." Once Sue's body got so far out of control, and her life was so desperately in disarray, that for three days she was on the verge of committing suicide.

Understandably, her severe and fluctuating symptoms were enormously disruptive to her life. For many months, she "made do," cutting back on activities, pacing them, delaying them, and so on. Thus her academic work gradually was put in abeyance. Her social life was radically curtailed, since she could never predict whether she would be able to keep commitments. She could call on friends to help with simple survival tasks, such as shopping for food. But it was embarrassing to do this repeatedly, so she often struggled to do this and other housekeeping tasks by herself. In short, because she was single and living alone, with minimal financial resources, many of the difficulties of everyday living were greatly magnified. Moreover, she lacked the psychological support that a cooperative spouse or other intimate generally provides. Nor did she have their counsel when making difficult and important decisions about medications, choice of physicians, whether it was wise to travel home at Christmas, how to handle her academic career—indeed, whether to go on living. Her arrangements to keep things going, let alone keep them together, were almost impossibly fragile. They remained so until her physical condition, for no apparent reason, became more or less stabilized about eighteen months later. Her savings exhausted, her academic work lagging far behind schedule, she settled for an administrative position in a large hospital, at least until her savings could be rebuilt.

Commentary

If the ill experience only mild instances of instability, especially if these are frequent, routines and strategies are developed for handling them. However, when the illness phases are very severe and prolonged, ordinary modes of managing illness and life become inadequate. One's immediate plans must be reformulated, modified, or discarded. Schedules of progress are shattered. Progress is nonlinear and difficult anyhow to evaluate. Experientially, victims of their own bodies—and sometimes of less than competent or astute physicians—live through a nightmare. Even if the instability is not quite so shattering, they may at the least become depressed. The goal of stabilization and a normal life recedes into the far distance. The overriding aim is just to stay in place and not become worse.

To manage instability, effective arrangements must be made. These cannot be merely those arrangements that sustain the stable phase of an illness or the usual round of everyday life. The arrangements during unstable phases are different— at the very least they are supplementary—and at best tend to be tentative, temporary, short-lived, and woefully fragile. During these unstable phases, the inadequacies of the current health care system can be seen with particular clarity, for the destabilized are relatively on their own then except for the usual clinical care.

The two case narratives illustrate these inadequacies; the gaps in the system to which they point are much the same. Both women were able to make certain necessary arrangements because they were fortunate enough to have sufficient funds to pay for certain services. They could also make other arrangements because one had a cooperative spouse and the other had cooperative friends. Neither could call on—or perhaps thought to call on—the health care system in *any* other way than for medical services.

Let us look at the monetary issue first, in terms of their arrangements for managing in the face of instability. Savings and income permitted them to purchase medical insurance; this paid for visits to physicians but not for all drugs. Psychiatric services were paid for out of pocket. So were the detoxification services. Another arrangement that apparently proved essential to Jan's regaining some stability was the remodeling of her house, but this was very expensive. Current health care institutional arrangements do not, by and large, cover such expenses, except perhaps for some of the costlier private insurance plans. Jan was additionally fortunate in that she worked at a university and so had no difficulties about her time away from teaching. Sue was also fortunate in being a student and so having no employer to satisfy; however, she spent her savings while making little progress in her academic career.

Both women also had to make arrangements to carry on their everyday obligations, especially housekeeping. They were fortunate in having no child-rearing duties to complicate matters: imagine if they had! Sue called on her friends, but she could resort to this informal network of emergency workers only occasionally. She had constantly to juggle these requests for assistance, being careful not to ask any one friend for help too frequently. Her increasing exhaustion forced her to abandon her dreams of earning a doctoral degree and pursuing an academic career. Jan had her husband to help, but since he happened to suffer from a bad back, with occasional unstable periods himself, the couple's division of labor left something to be desired. In any event, this particular marriage, which had not been tested by long years of living together, was pushed to the limit by Jan's frequent and long periods of instability. Marital stress and physical exhaustion increased; eventually, the marriage broke up.

How might the health care system have offered housekeeping and other home care services to these women? We must conclude either that no institutional services were available or that they did not find them. If certain services were actually available, they were so invisible and insufficient, and the agency system so fragmented, that they were not realistically available to these women. Sue was a nurse, studying at an outstanding school of nursing, with nurses as friends—but none of this helped her find useful services; nor did her physician focus on anything but her acute care. One can empathize with the physicians of both women, struggling without much success with genuinely difficult cases, but the typical physician-specialist has little idea of what it is like to live with such instability. Those physicians who know feel helpless before it.

Next, let us look at how both women coordinated their medical care, without assistance from the health care system. In brief, they had to do this themselves, although Jan had her husband's help. The current fragmented state of medical services contributes to this situation of the ill and their families. The plight of the unstable ill is rendered additionally difficult and the consequences especially stressful if, like Sue, they suffer from more than one chronic illness, with the consequent need to monitor several different regimens. They must monitor the side effects not only of each drug but also of their interactions; in Jan's case, medication may have had very deleterious long-term and cumulative effects. These ill people also need to make assessments about which regimens are working and which are not, when and how to report their assessments to the physician, and so on.

The health care system offers neither counsel nor psychological support to people like this during the worst of their travail. If it does offer these services, they are essentially unavailable to most of the potential clients. Furthermore, given the well-described bureaucratic maze that both clients and health workers report with respect to such home care services, how can these frequently exhausted people be expected to discover where those services are and for which ones they qualify? This situation is especially characteristic of ill people who live alone with no energetic intimate or kin to do the necessary investigative work. Sadly, not even self-help groups are adapted to serve the severely destabilized; these groups are designed mainly to help keep people stable (as with diabetic groups) or to give psychological support (as with cancer groups).

In sum, these cases suggest that people who are undergoing unstable trajectory phases—when the instability is particularly severe or long-term—are not well served by the health care system. It is designed primarily for the acute and immediate postacute, or rehabilitation, periods. However, it is not geared to serve its clients if their conditions later become unstable. During periods of severe destabilization, everyone is defeated—the ill, their intimates and friends, the professionals themselves—by a combination of extensive physical destabilization and a health care system that fails to deliver resources via effective institutional arrangements.

Summary

Unstable phases are causally linked both with changes in physiological status and with various behavioral and social conditions. Among them are carelessly kept regimens, poor monitoring, inadequate illness management, inappropriate environmental conditions, and the miscalculation of physical capacities. These unstable periods should not be conceived of in terms of acute care nor as wholly a matter of medical management. The more unstable a person becomes, the more probable it is that work arrangements will crumble and resources necessary for the return to stability will dwindle. This contributes to further instability. In extreme instances, physicians may be unable to hit upon the right treatments.

During unstable periods, the inadequacies of the health care system are particularly visible, for the destabilized are on their own except for the usual types of clinical care. The women in both case illustrations were fortunate in being able to make or continue necessary work arrangements, but for the single woman these became increasingly fragile. Neither thought to call on the health care system in any other way than for clinical services. Financial costs were a burden, though both women had moderate financial means. Services like housekeeping assistance, home care, counseling, and coordination of management work, including medical management, were not thought of either by the women themselves or by their physicians. In such cases of extended instability, it is doubtful whether long-term services are even available unless they are paid for by the ill themselves. Thus, the conditions for destabilizing the chronically ill also include the failures of a health care system that does not reach people moving into or already in unstable phases.

9

∗ ∗ ∗ ∗ ∗

Facing Deterioration

In the trajectory phase of deterioration, physiological or physical capacity, and usually functional ability, decrease. Different types of social arrangements and services are necessary for early, middle, and late stages of deterioration. During the early period, the ill may need assistance in coming to terms with the current disabilities and their anxiety about future problems. In the middle stage, they may have to retire from a job, cut back on their housekeeping work, or hire someone to do the heavier chores. They probably cannot yet qualify for home care, however, even if they were to think of requesting it. In the later stages of deterioration, the ill can profit from a battery of home care services, yet they may be in no financial condition to pay for many, or any, of these.

The deteriorating ill, whatever the degree of their disability, have made a host of social arrangements for carrying on despite their illness. Yet even a slight change in their physical condition can upset some crucial aspect of their arrangements. A major change can wreak havoc. Conversely, a change in the arrangements or in the resources supporting them (such as the death of a spouse, a divorce, or the marriage of a caretaking daughter) can drastically affect the ill person's ability to stay relatively stable. Further physical decline results. In any event, each further physical decline necessitates rearrangements. If these are not effective, illness management suffers. The aim of the arrangements and rearrangements is to maintain as much stability as possible—the stability not only of the illness but of the flow of life, at as high a level of quality as possible.

The three cases presented in this chapter illustrate some of these points. Like many of the cases in preceding chapters, they also bring out major policy issues that pertain especially to the vulnerability of arrangements, the difficulty of being knowledgeable about health services, the problem of accessibility to them, the agency maze that compounds these difficulties, and the gaps in American health care services.

The Karls: End of the Trail

Picture a baseball game in the ninth inning. The bases are loaded; the score is tied. Coming up is a wicked trio of powerful batters. But the pitcher is weary and there is no replacement. This is precisely the situation of countless elderly men and women whose ill partners have deteriorated so alarmingly that death is close, although not immediate, and the couple now have only meager financial and physical resources to see them through their final years.

Their plight cannot simply be blamed on their thoughtlessness in not preparing for these contingent circumstances. For those are related not merely to individuals' abilities to save and plan for their last decades, but to some of the more inhumane features of American society. Usually these couples—even those of the middle classes—have had their financial resources depleted by years of paying for medical care attendant on the chronic illness of one or both partners. Most medical insurance plans do not adequately cover illnesses that bring considerable and even impossibly heavy expenses over the long term. Nor do the plans pay for the various home services that would relieve spouses, who earlier might have had enough energy to be caretakers and homemakers but now are physically wearing out—if indeed they remain free from illness themselves. True, Medicare, Medicaid, and various social services are theoretically available. We shall see their inadequacies and actual inaccessibility highlighted in the case of the Karls, an elderly couple. We have only the wife's account because the husband's advanced emphysema precluded his being interviewed.

The husband, formerly in good health, developed angina at the age of seventy. At seventy-three he became legally blind (he can see but can't drive) and developed emphysema. Now, at seventy-nine, he is so debilitated by his emphysema that he depends on continuous oxygen therapy. He is also on a catheter for a prostate problem following an unsuccessful prostate operation. He has been hospitalized for either the prostate or the emphysema thirteen or fourteen times, four or five times in an emergency condition.

The Karls are a childless couple whose remaining kin do not live in the same region. Like many other elderly people, they are "at a point where so many . . . friends are gone. . . . The men are gone and the women are sick." She herself takes her husband to the hospital via ambulance or taxi when he needs to go; "I have no family or anyone to call on. I have taken him there and have not known whether I was going to be able to get him there or not." When she reads his bodily signs, "sometimes it has been hard for me to know if it is time to take him because I am here alone." But the potential mistakes are frightening: "That time he told me, 'I feel queer, oh I feel so queer.' Then I looked back and thought, well he has been different, just a general weakness I guess. It was a good thing because he had to go into intensive care."

Because of the characteristics of his disablement and his regimen requirements, she has to work very hard—quite aside from all the monitoring and assessing of his condition that she does, and all of her household tasks besides. We can get some sense of the amount of her work from her description of an ordinary day:

> I can't believe how you can be so busy. The days are very much the same. I get up around seven and get breakfast and his four medicines. Then fix the bronkosol for his treatment. He can hold it himself, but I have to watch so he doesn't go back to sleep.

The attendant does it when he is there. He gets four treatments daily. I check on the medicines. If it's getting low, I call the drugstore. The routines are pretty much the same every day. I haven't always had help: on and off. We had to stop for a while because of our finances. Now he is so bedridden, there's no choice. I used to help him bathe and shave, before. Now when it's impossible for him to help himself, we use an attendant. On the attendant's days off, I'm lax about bathing him. Sometimes I don't shave him, if no one is visiting. The medications are four times a day, and he takes about five different ones.

They pay the attendant five dollars an hour, and somehow she manages when the attendant is not there. They have meals on wheels four times a week. When friends ask her if she likes that, she says, "Not exactly, but it is better than trying to cook at night." She's too tired. For lunch, "I just make sandwiches." In effect, "I'm on call all the time." Sometimes she gets so tired that she lashes out at him. For eight months now—after some months of using a wheelchair at home—he has had to stay in bed unless the attendant is there to get him up and later to put him back to bed. "Physically I can't get him up anymore." As he gets worse, and emergency visits to the hospital become more frequent, the psychological pressure on her increases. "For a while I was awfully nervous and thought maybe I should go and see a psychiatrist." But then she reasoned, "Well, there is no point in that because I know what is doing it. Just the stress and the financial problems getting awfully bad."

A while ago, their income was about $950 per month, which seemed to be sufficient. Then the rent began to be raised, so they have had to sell some government bonds. She had read "somewhere" about a rent supplement, but does not know where it is or how to get it. She called and got some "pointers, but what I need is more personal help and some finances. Other people can't do that." Medicare pays their hospital bills, "but it doesn't pay extra doctors they bring in, and the extras." During one hospitalization, the husband fractured a vertebra turning over in bed and had to have a bone specialist visit him. "The big problem is that Medicare and Blue Cross make mistakes, and you have to call them up and get them on the phone, and you can't get them." The medical bills "just pile up; I don't know if I have gotten all that we should or not. . . . With his medical bills he should be on Medi-Cal, but both spouses would have to be on it," and they "have too much [savings] to be eligible." When she herself had to be hospitalized for Parkinsonian symptoms, she put her husband in a nursing home for eleven days. The bill was "over three thousand dollars."

They had always saved for these days; now they are reduced to trying to stay off welfare. They had earlier talked about his having eventually to live in a nursing home, but the $1,500 per month that it would cost is well beyond their means. Previously, she thought that if and when "something happened to him," she could buy into a place for the elderly "like the Heritage; that was very lovely, but now I won't be able to."

Her husband says it is all right to leave him alone in the apartment for a while, to shop or go to the bank, but she can't leave him for very long. She is afraid of an earthquake or a fire, and she worries that he might need a bedpan. One friend has asked why she doesn't ask for help at her church. "It's hard for me to ask people to do anything for me." This reluctance extends even to a couple who said they would be glad to help.

Being alone so much, and because of the deaths of their closest friends, she gets lonely. When the telephone rings, it makes her happy: "Somebody is thinking about us," and talking on the phone "helps to relieve the loneliness." Her husband and she had been quite sociable, and of course she misses that sociability. Nowadays, she does not talk about her troubles to her friends, but "just to get my mind off myself helps." She adds that in fact she is worried about what she can talk about other than her own pressing daily problems.

The strain of the last years particularly, plus her increasingly "chronic fatigue," makes her occasionally more irritable toward her husband and sometimes "very depressed. Why is all this happening? Why does old age have to be this way? Then I try to snap out of it because there is really nothing you can do about it.'' Sometimes she goes into the kitchen to cry so that her husband can't hear her. Yet occasionally she talks to him about how worried she is. ''He doesn't worry about it, he says 'Oh, it will be all right. Don't worry.''' But, she adds, ''He is probably worried himself.'' In any event, she does not talk to other people about any of this, because ''they would say I am neurotic.''

Yet ''it's hard when you look at your husband and think of what he used to be.'' Still, he remains ''very affectionate,'' and wants to be kissed a lot. She loves him but wouldn't want to die herself if he dies (she is crying as she admits this). Now ''it's just a matter of prolonging his life. Sometimes he says he would like to die, then other times he is afraid he might. He says 'except for you I would like to go.' He says he would like to stay so he can help me, but he can't help me. Maybe there is something I can do, he says. I asked him what kind of a funeral he would like, if he would like to be cremated. He said, no, he would like to be buried next to his sister.'' Whenever he is hospitalized, at least this allows her ''to get out and do things [for] it's boring to just sit there all day.'' She gets tired, she worries, she is near the end of their trail, knowing full well, as she says, that ''at this age it is not going to be very long anyway.'' In short, this couple, without health, resources, or savings, is in the grip of events and feels power-less to stop them.

Commentary

These are middle-income people; they were never affluent, but until their early seventies they lived comfortably, with rel-ative financial security. Despite Medicare and private medical insurance, his prolonged illness and frequent medical expenses have reduced their savings drastically. Moreover, despite the actual availability of other health and social services, such middle-class couples often do not know how to find these services, nor are they actually discovered by the servicing agencies. By contrast, lower-class families might well be more savvy about such services or more likely to be found by the agencies. The independence of middle-class people can become a liability when the basis for that independence begins to crumble.

When, however, middle-class persons are relatively aggressive about researching available services, they can find them. After all, even the Yellow Pages of the phone book are of some help. Yet their physicians are far from knowledgeable about such matters, and apparently are often unlikely to proffer information about such services, while many couples are shy about pressuring physicians or nurses for such information. Their friends are no more likely to know of the existence of these services or how to go about finding them. Pride is also a barrier to asking for help in finding services or to directly requesting them. These Americans are raised to be independent, and they are often deeply ashamed, even terrified, to be thrust into the position of receiving free aid—to fall into the class of "paupers" who are on welfare.

Insofar as they may be fortunate enough to be on Medicare or solvent enough to carry private medical insurance, at least some of their medical and financial burden is lifted. Yet, as this elderly wife tells us, for the physically weary (and often financially rather uneducated), the difficulties of figuring out medical bills are staggering and anxiety-provoking. Trying to get mistakes "straightened out" by the authorities is time-consuming and frustrating. The system sometimes seems surrealistic to them, apparently designed both to cheat them and to thwart efforts to get the correct answers. These bedeviled people surely need help in their bookkeeping and in reaching the proper authorities. This is perhaps especially true for the wives whose husbands had previously been largely responsible for the family's financial affairs. However, no such help is available to them. Meanwhile, all of this anxiety about finances is added to the tremendous stress of anxiety over the illness itself, the burdens of managing both illness and other work, and, sometimes, the stress of a dissolving marital relationship.

For such aging couples, the physical stability of an ill partner becomes increasingly problematic. One reason is the continued course of the illness; another is the development of additional illnesses, which may add to the burdens cumulatively through their physiological interaction. If further physical deterioration results in even the slightest negative changes in the ill person's condition, shifts in current arrangements are called for. Each permanent drop in physical condition thus necessitates readjustments in daily life: the person is now bedridden, or can no longer drive or walk up steps and slopes, or must eat only low-salt food. These rearrangements, if they are to be successful, must rest on good judgment, and perhaps on ingenuity, concerning spheres of life other than the medical. The rearrangements involve issues of bodily mobility, housekeeping chores, financial changes, social relationships, marital relationships, even legal matters. The rearrangements also involve matters of deep identity. All of this is crowding in precisely when the couples are most likely to find themselves increasingly isolated from helping friends and relatives. Unquestionably, they need counsel, guidance, and sometimes additional resources to institute the needed rearrangements.

The continued deterioration of an ill spouse, and its impact on various spheres of life, can cause great psychological strain on the well partner. As researchers, we have seen instances when the toll of the daily burden and the psychological wear and tear resulted in heavy drinking; each night, the exhausted and dazed caretaker would escape into befuddled sleep. Whether handled through liquor, bouts of anger against the ill partner, or some other mechanism, the strain of continued and increasing physical deterioration can result in a spiral of increasing marital discord. Inevitably, the increasing distress of either partner brings reactions from the other, and heightens the other's stress too. The ill may wonder despairingly, as did one man, whether it is fair to the other spouse to prolong their own living. Presumably, some find their way out of that seemingly no-exit situation.

This dismal picture of the elderly sick is relieved by a continued marital closeness, as with Mr. and Mrs. Karl, or at least by a continued sense of obligation. Marital commitments,

whether from love or obligation, keep the couples going somehow, but increasingly the odds are against them in this fateful
game. Why is this so, other than the increasing difficulty or
devastation of cumulative illness? As the well partners become
older, they too are likely to develop chronic illnesses, and so
are less able to carry the burdens of managing medical care or
doing household tasks. Precisely when the partners need a greater
amount of energy to cope with increasing burdens, their energy
lessens. Often, too, as we have seen, their financial resources
decrease as medical costs and other expenses increase. Programs
like Medicare and Social Security are supposed to handle this
situation, but of course they do not at all fully handle it, whether
financially, medically, or in terms of counseling about psychological, social, and legal matters. Furthermore, the American
safety net for medical care, supposedly constituted by the various
mechanisms of governmental funding and services, does not
much affect the need for end-of-the-trail care; elderly people like
Mr. and Mrs. Karl cannot rely on such aid when their own funds
are insufficient to purchase nursing home care.

In reflecting on the sad tales told by such couples, one
conclusion is evident. While medical problems may be at the
center of difficult life circumstances, health policy must take the
full range of these life circumstances into consideration as con-
stituting a multiple interacting set. Any health policy that does
not will be in large measure ineffective.

People like the Karls need counsel about a range of difficult circumstances and about services some of which they can
afford and some not; some available, if only they knew about
them, and some theoretically available but essentially inaccessible
to them. It is not so much direct financing that such couples
need to ease their burdens—although a little of that can surely
help—but counseling services. Their lifelong sense of independence is both their great strength and a cause of their vulnerability. They are vulnerable in the face of severe, prolonged illness
that has depleted their resources and energies, and in the face
of a health system that has more or less failed them in all but
strictly clinical ways.

Mrs. Johnson: How Little May Be Needed

This is the story of an eighty-three-year-old woman, blessed with a devoted and highly educated son, but living a continent apart from him when her immediate social support had vanished and her physical condition had almost reached zero. Their experiences point up the following policy issues:

1. How close to the edge of social and psychological disaster, and medical disaster too, the elderly sometimes live; how precarious the social arrangements can be that stand between relatively normal, satisfying living and disaster
2. What happens to them during medical and social psychological crises when their families live at a distance
3. The difficulties that even health professionals can have in finding their way through the agency maze when seeking services for their own kin
4. The gaps in health care resources and social services for these very deteriorated ill people
5. How little it can take to restore the delicate balance to their lives if the right arrangements are made or if services are found—and what kind they are, and should be, under a more effective health care system

Mrs. Johnson lived in Florida in her own small house. Although she suffered from several chronic conditions, including deteriorating kidneys, an abdominal aneurysm, and hypertension, nevertheless she was quite active. She shopped, did some housework, visited friends, and was a respected member of her church community. Living with her in an intimate relationship was a middle-aged daughter. Between them, to quote her son, Tom, "a certain kind of life-style was developed around the two of them being mutually responsible for each other." Her son, a long-time resident of California, visited his mother occasionally and telephoned frequently. Tom has a master's degree in social work and has worked in a major medical center for many years as a social worker.

About six months before his mother's death, Tom returned from an extended stay in Florida, where he had been because of a medical emergency in his mother's life. Tom noted that she had done very well for the past seven or eight years. However, during this period he had been concerned about "what will happen to momma if something happens." Something eventually did happen: the death of her daughter, two years before our interview with Tom. After that, his mother's physical condition deteriorated rapidly. She had a heart attack about one year later, and since then her memory had become somewhat impaired and she had developed an ulcer. She had understood the significance of the aneurysm but refused to have surgery: "She wanted to die with all that she had originally been given."

After the daughter's death, Tom had talked with his mother's physician, who believed that basically she was doing all right. "In the meantime, there were always friends coming to visit from the church, so there was a periodic check on her. I sort of put the responsibility on them in the sense that they saw her as often as they did. So they cued me in to what they saw."

At one point, on hearing her speech, Tom thought she had suffered a stroke. However, "each time I'd gone home I was impressed with all the medication that had been prescribed. I was concerned about how she could juggle all those medicines." Her tendency, he thought, was to relieve her symptoms quickly, since she was "a bit hypochondriacal. So I wondered [and] talked to the physicians." They thought something was wrong; her heart at the last examination had seemed larger, possibly from some kind of cardiac distress after a recent heart attack.

Tom talked with her on the telephone immediately afterward several times. A friend of his mother's agreed to spend the night with her. To Tom, who talked to her on the phone that night, it seemed that as the night progressed, she was becoming worse. In the morning, another friend stayed briefly with her. Yet the longer he talked with his mother, the worse she seemed to get. "Then I suggested she hang up the telephone, because I wanted to call somebody else to see if they could come over. She never did that, the phone never disconnected. So I called a friend, and she said she'd hospitalize her if I gave permission. Meantime I called the physician, and he said, 'Fine.'"

Tom talked later with this physician, who had discovered that Mrs. Johnson had inadvertently overdosed herself. However, "he didn't think he'd be willing to discharge her home alone. I raised questions about the medicine, having talked previously to him about it." The physician had earlier asked her to bring all of her medications to him, and after examining them discarded a great number. After that, she had been overdosing herself with a new pain medication. The physician told Tom that he needed to think seriously about an alternative to her living alone—perhaps a nursing home. She was currently eligible under Medicare for postsurgery home care, including visiting nurses, a nurses' aide, and homemaker services. The physician had authorized those services because this was possible during a posthospital period.

As Tom explained, "I had to think about the long term. So I went home, trying to point out to her the options that existed as well as the options that didn't exist. That if her grandchildren weren't living [in Florida] they might as well not be there. . . . I asked if she didn't want to live with me, what about close by? But she said no, for as she had said before she preferred to live and die at home. In her own house if possible." The doctor had talked about nursing homes to her, but "in no way did she want to go to a nursing home." The physician said he could provide her with home care as long as there was a medical need, "but once that need was abated, she would then be left on her own. . . . The only time then she could get home care again was if her condition became exacerbated again." Tom and the physician then talked about "what we could do to keep her at home."

Tom remained in Florida and for two weeks carefully checked all the Florida Welfare Department publications. He began this search "hopeful that I would find something." What he found was that despite Senator Claude Pepper's energetic efforts on behalf of the elderly, Florida was "still behind in many ways [in not having] some really good support programs. The welfare department could only offer emergency types of care."

As for proprietary care, that was almost completely impossible, financially speaking. Mrs. Johnson's Social Security payments were "something like $300 a month. And my mother had only a limited income." Tom contributed $100 monthly for her support, but "I couldn't document that or it would be taken from her Social Security grant." Returning later to Florida, he interviewed people at various agencies. The proprietary costs would be $2,200 per month, covering only five days each week; he would have to negotiate for weekend care, which would cost an additional $1,300 per month. "In the meantime, I'm still working with her, and a social worker who continues to give me support in looking for resources, but does not see herself as a resource. And I guess toward the end of the second week I started packing for home."

Earlier, when his sister was ill and in the hospital, she had arranged for her friends and her mother's friends to drop by the house to "check up on things." Some of them still come by every day, and have keys to her house. Three years before, Tom had set up in the house a device whereby, if his mother ran into trouble at night, she could get some sort of response from one friend "by pressing this [button]. . . . She had a certain kind of support there. And people were very good about getting her to the physician when she couldn't do it on her own." He had also arranged for meals on wheels because he did not trust her to cook regularly. "I thought I had set up a pretty good network as well as resources. But here we were talking about something more intense and of longer duration, and the public agencies didn't seem to have it. Plus my own resources were limited. So I felt I had to do something to manage" the situation.

He interviewed a number of people as potential caretakers without success. Some could come for a couple of hours a day, but none could come on a permanent basis "at a cost that I could absorb." Then, suddenly, they had a stroke of good fortune. A friend from church called, saying she knew of someone who had worked for the past ten years as a companion for an elderly couple and who was now available. When this woman came to the house, "the first thing she did when she walked in was to shake my mother's hand and kiss her on the cheek. And my mother said, 'She's the one, this is the one I want!' She's been there since. I've gone home once since then and been impressed not only with how well they get along but the change in my mother's overall situation.'' His mother was still clinically at risk and was hospitalized once, ''but the affect and quality of her life has so changed.'' In the past, whenever he had called from California during the day, he could be pretty certain he would find his mother at home. ''Now six times out of ten I won't.'' The companion had a car, so they went out. Recently his mother went shopping in three different places, and walked everywhere without her walker.

The companion charged fifteen dollars per day, ''which I can't claim because she's on Social Security. Both my mother and she are Social Security recipients so both would be in great jeopardy of losing their grants if I attempted to claim this.'' His mother's condition, he judged, now ''is as stable as it can be.'' Yet he still worried about his mother's death, ''and we've talked about that.'' She had arranged for various relatives to visit, and was waiting for one more: ''When [that relative] comes, she knows it will be time, she says, to go. But this was before Mrs. Jones came into the scene and into her life. And when we talk about that now, she recognizes that death is real but she's not afraid. I don't think she's ever been afraid. . . . Now she's visiting friends, she's resumed her work in the church.'' Six months later, after carefully closing off her kinship and social life, his mother died. It is important for understanding how relatively stable her life had become to know that as she neared her death, this appreciative woman was preparing her son for the time when she would no longer be alive.

Commentary

This case has at least five important policy implications. First of all, it graphically illustrates how close to the edge of social, psychological, and physiological disaster the elderly sometimes live. The first two can help to precipitate the third. As people's bodies deteriorate, their lives hang in increasingly delicate balance. Their lives as biological beings as well as human beings are endangered when their supportive arrangements become fragile. Many a fragile elderly person has been thrust abruptly into a nursing home, often to die there speedily, because a spouse died, or because she almost set her apartment on fire when cooking.

Mrs. Johnson went rapidly downhill both physiologically and socially after losing her daughter. Tom managed to restore stability in her life, to give her a chance to resume a relatively active communal church life, and quite possibly to slow down her physical decline. If Mrs. Jones had left his mother, he would have had to begin all over again to assemble the necessary resources for maintaining his mother's life.

A second issue pertains to close kin living at a distance. Tom's story sheds some light on how support can be mustered even when committed kin live far away. However, kinfolk would have to be very devoted, very committed, to persist for as long as he did and to act in such careful detail. Tom was, of course, unusual in having extensive professional knowledge and experience; certainly, too, there was his empathy and his sensitivity to his mother's wishes and style of life. He also understood the central importance of maintaining and strengthening a social network around his mother—a supportive set of arrangements. His mother was also extremely fortunate in having as friends people who were less feeble than she. Indeed, many elderly often discover they have no friends at all, or none on whom they can count in emergencies. Many welfare and health practitioners do not understand the importance of a social network; others feel themselves powerless when attempting to build or strengthen networks for certain clients. At the other extreme, sometimes kin do not properly appreciate how essential a parent's long-standing informal networks are for his or her quality of life. They may even shatter these relationships when insisting that sick parents move away from their own homes. Yet survival considerations often take precedence over quality of life in such decision making. The policy issue here is what might be done to encourage adult children and other kin who do not live close by to give greater support to the ill person. What financial and other organizational arrangements might further this kind of family assistance and coordination?

A third issue raised by Tom's story is the difficulty that relatively untutored people, or even educated ones, can have finding their way through the so-called agency maze. Even Tom, an experienced social worker, finds himself having to spend two weeks intensively searching for whatever services might be available. The fourth issue is the huge and consequential gaps in those services. If you have little or no money, then you get no proprietary care. If, as is often the case, there are few or no social services—services applicable to your case, for otherwise they might just as well be located on the moon—then you are simply out of luck. In the United States, you are dependent on luck: it may bring a savior like Mrs. Jones, or it may take you to the worst sort of nursing home. It may also lead to a quick death.

The fifth issue raised by the Johnsons' story is how very little it takes to restore the delicate balance to the ill person's life. If the appropriate resources and services are found, they can be tremendously effective. It is worthwhile to emphasize that these are not necessarily costly. Mrs. Johnson's story points to the usefulness of moving policy in two directions. The first is to avoid bifurcating social and medical services in conception and organization. These services must be organically connected. The second is to extend home care funding to conscientious helpers. Even if they are not educated or trained at high levels, they can be crucial for certain kinds of tasks done for the ill and their families. These include not simply custodial but also medical services, such as monitoring symptoms, giving injections, and doing other simple clinical procedures. Consider what might happen if home care funding included even more highly trained professionals who were both conscientious and, like Mrs. Jones, rich in expressive gesture and action.

Mrs. Stutz: Government
Policy and the Human Predicament

The next case is about a husband with Alzheimer's disease and his caretaking wife. Only the aspects of their lives that pertain to their financial hardships will be emphasized. As is well recognized, so-called catastrophic illness can lead to great financial difficulties for families. Some of our previous cases have tangentially illustrated this human predicament; in this case, we focus on government's role in it. In the United States, for a variety of reasons, federal and state governments have been extremely loath to build a financial safety net under people who are facing impoverishment because of illness. This segment of our population's physical and financial plight is deliberately ignored by governmental agencies that are perfectly capable of easing their financial burdens. We say ''perfectly capable'' meaning that this could be done if the appropriate organizational machinery were mandated and in place, or if the existing machinery were more effectively operated.

Sometimes it is not easy for those who apply for agency services to know whether the agency system is defective or legislative rules are at the heart of their difficulties with accessibility of and qualification for services. In any event, the health care system appears heartless: it is only a question of whether the cruelties it unquestionably inflicts are due to bureaucratic inefficiencies or calculated refusal to bear the supportive costs. Ultimately, there is not much question that even the agency mazes encountered by the ill and their kin result mainly from either shortsighted or closefisted governmental policies.

The Stutzes are a relatively well-to-do couple in their mid sixties. Mr. Stutz was an engineer until he retired eleven years ago because of the debilitating effects of Alzheimer's. Over the years, his decline has followed the usual bizarre pattern now recognized by anyone who has read the descriptions of this disease in the mass media. The strain on his wife has also followed the pattern for increasingly burdened and psychologically distressed caretakers. The Stutzes' adult children do not live at home, so Mrs. Stutz is the sole caretaker.

In order to portray the experiences of the caretaker with regard to the disastrous combination of extreme deterioration and governmental inaction, we quote at length from her story. She is telling us about her attempts to stay afloat financially in the excerpts given below.

I thought, I can't handle this. I've got to put him in a nursing home for a while anyway. . . . I started putting the wheels in motion—calling people, talking to this one, talking to that one, got all kinds of bad advice. People told me Medicare would pay for the first three months in a nursing home. Professionals told me this. Professionals told me I could wait and put him on Medicaid until he was in the hospital, that somebody would do it from the hospital. They said in no way. If he's got somebody that can do it for him, we don't go to the hospital. So I had to go. The day that I put him in a nursing home in the morning I went to Medicaid in the afternoon. I talked to an agency that places patients in nursing homes . . . and she's the one who said, you won't get him on Medicare. Medicare is going around checking everybody. They are not paying out the way they used to. And she said, he's not going to be paid for you. You are going to have to figure out something else. So, there I was putting him in a nursing home and not knowing which way things were going, and no real financial resources. But anyway, I did get him put on Medicaid. He went in as a private patient the first month because I was told it would be easier that way. And then he got on Medicaid.

Oh, another thing. I never put down Alzheimer's on anything. We were told not to do that. If there were some other health problem, use that because the insurance companies and all these other places will not pay for Alzheimer's. They consider it a mental problem—we don't pay for that, physical problems we do. So I would put down Parkinson's-Dementia. Who knows whether it's Parkinson's or dementia? In fact, I've often wondered lately because he seems to be going on long and strong.

. . . With Medicaid you're walking a tightrope. I went to Medicaid to see if I could get a part-

time job and keep the money in addition to—I get
part of his Social Security—and so I am under the
thumb of Medicaid even though I don't get Medicaid [myself] because he [does]. . . . Money is a real
problem when you have a patient on Medicaid. I
mean, look at all the years that he has been on
disability. Those were the years he would have been
so productive, the years that he had to quit working. Anyway, I have been battling with Medicaid
trying to find out if I can go to work under this new
law that was just passed last year, where you have
effective financial divorce. . . .

I found out that Medicaid had put in for
medication that I had to pay for within the last two
to three years. There were certain things Medicaid
would not cover. If you had a skin rash, which John
has constantly, they should use talcum powder and
a certain kind of soap, and if they had skin rashes—
tough—then the family pays for it. And so I paid
for all those.

I don't even want to deal with Medicaid.
They are just a nightmare. They took John off
Medicaid in September for just a few days through
a misunderstanding and it still isn't straightened
out. What happened was that he turned sixty-five
last April. OK, he went off disability. He was supposed to go on regular retirement with Johnson [his
former employer] and I had a letter dated two years
before—I kept all this stuff, it drives me crazy—
saying . . . what will happen. He will go off disability, he will go onto his pension—so nothing happened. I didn't find out until I got my bank balance
that I didn't get the money that month. Here I
thought I had, you know, more money than I
thought I had in the bank, I'd gotten it for one-
third of the month, until he turned sixty-five. So
I called up Connecticut General long-distance and
they said . . . and I said, I was told that this would

happen . . . oh, no, no, you have to write and initiate it. . . . And I said, but you always sent me
so many forms before, well in advance. . . . Well,
there's been a change in policy . . . which I think
means that if you don't have enough smarts you
don't get it. So anyway, it took six months for his
pension to come through. . . . So that came through
in the fall . . . and I got a lump sum. So I called
up Medicaid—you have to report within ten days
any change—whatever happens to you, any change
in finances—so I reported to them. So they said,
oh well, we will have to consider that income for
you. . . . I think I'm going to wind up with well
over $2,000 that I owe them. I think they are go-
ing to take the whole thing away but they haven't
told me what they are doing. In the meantime, they
have taken John off Medicaid because you have to
fill [out forms]. . . . They are forever sending you
letters, do this within ten days or your patient will
be taken off. Well, what I had done, my mother
had moved in with me. I had to write a letter—she
had to write a letter. I had to tell them how much
she was paying me and board and the whole thing.
They took some of her board and were putting it
toward John at the nursing home. They said, they
told me, that a family of four should be able to live
for $111 per person per month. I said, will you tell
me where—I'll rush there—can you believe that?

So anyway, I had written all that out. When
I had filled out the form for John in September—
you have to do it every year—it said, you know,
who is living at your house. So I wrote, mother—
and then I thought, No, I had put John's name and
then I would put mother-in-law. . . . Well, the gal
didn't figure it out. She thought I had another person living at the house paying me board that I
hadn't reported . . . so she cut John off Medicaid.
In the meantime, I am still waiting. . . .

I wrote a letter. I have a letter from Lincoln. I called up Lincoln about this. I said, you know, under this new law I think I should be able to go to work and keep my money. . . . I finally got to see the supervisor after two months of phoning. I wrote a letter in June, got a letter back from this man that I talked to in Lincoln who was with Medicaid. He seemed to think I could do it. I finally got to see this supervisor in August and she said, well, you will be a test case. I said, all I want to do is to go out and get about $300 per month and keep it and put it in the bank so that I will be able to buy a new roof and what's needed for the house. So she said, oh well, you can keep your money . . . the thing is we give you $509 now to live on out of John's money and she said, if you earn $500 you can keep it—we'd only give you $9. I said, will you tell me the incentive in going to work? I said, I need to save some money. I need a large sum. A new roof costs $5,000. . . . Well, we will make it a test case. . . . Well, I have not heard it to this day.

When John was taken off Medicaid, of course naturally I got on the phone as soon as possible and I talked to my social worker and she finally said, well, write a letter. . . . I said, this is not my mother-in-law—my mother-in-law is dead, this is my mother. I wrote to you a year ago about that, you've got it all in your file. . . . Well, write this letter, do this, do that, and we'll put him back on. Let's see, he didn't get back on the computer till December. This was the beginning of September that this happened.

You are a nonentity. You are a third-class citizen. You are nobody when you are dealing with the government and with bureaucracy—it is one of the most frustrating things that I have ever encountered. I didn't think there could be anything much worse than having a spouse with Alzheimer's disease and dementia and watching them go slowly down the tubes. . . . But I'll tell you there is one thing worse and this is having a spouse with Alzheimer's disease who is on Medicaid under the old rules. It is terrible. You just can't imagine. In fact, my brother-in-law said to me, he said, you've got more restrictions in your life than the fellow that shot the Stanford professor—that just got out of jail. He said, he can go where he wants to and he doesn't have this, that, and the other thing to do and report within ten days and you know. . . . The whole system is just totally frustrating. It is not realistic.

I've had professionals, and I won't quote who they are, but I've had several professionals who are in the field, who are dealing with this all of the time, who have said—forget what you learned years ago. You just take your resources—of course you do it well in advance—but you hide any money that you have with a branch over here—you can do it all quite legally but you have to know in advance.

Right, this is not quite such a problem now that they have this new law. . . . There are people out there with a lot of money who had planned for a lovely retirement and they would have to put their patient in a nursing home and spend all their money down to $3,000 for a couple. . . . You can't have life insurance . . . you have to cash in your life insurance. This is not true in all states but it is true in Nebraska. . . . John has term, fortunately, with Johnson, nothing like he had before, just enough to bury him probably . . . but yes, I've cashed in my life insurance. If I hadn't I would have had to spend it on the nursing home for him. I cashed it in because I wasn't getting any money on it and I was trying to be a little smart and I put it where it would get a little more interest. . . . Well, then we had to spend it anyway, you know, to get John in the nursing home. . . .

So, it's really a nightmare . . . and I'm at a
stage where I would love to go back to work.

Mrs. Stutz finally managed to get her husband permanently into a nursing home, but only by claiming that he had
Parkinson's disease. By dint of shrewd maneuvering, and probably some insider advice, she managed to outwit Medicaid and
thus to keep ownership of her house, even though Medicaid paid
for the nursing home expense.

Commentary

Let us not focus unduly on Mrs. Stutz's frustration and
anger at the governmental process, nor on her sense of being
humiliated and given the runaround by inefficient and heartless
personnel. More important are the details of how this governmental process is seen through her eyes. While her experiences
may add up to an extreme case, at least some of them are shared
by countless other hapless caretakers or by the ill themselves
when they seek help and guidance. Stated briefly, here is a partial
list of her points:

1.   People tell you different things about some of the rules.
      There is a lot of confusion about this. If you are lucky, you
      find someone who knows what is really so.
2.   When there is a new rule or law, those who should know
      whether it applies to me in fact do not.
3.   You have to discover yourself what Medicaid pays for and
      what it doesn't. Then you also discover that they make
      mistakes—some of which cost you money—as well as causing confusion in your life and your plans. They can even
      make the major mistake of deciding erroneously that your
      husband should be sent home from the nursing home.
4.   When you want to work, you also discover that Medicaid
      won't let you do that if you want them to help fund your
      husband's case. Yet you also need to work in order to get
      some of your own expenses paid.
5.   When you deal with Medicaid personnel they can be confused and confusing, impersonal, bureaucratic.

6. You have to outwit Medicaid by canny maneuvering. Insider professionals sometimes help you by suggesting how to do that.
7. Meanwhile, your life is further complicated by having to juggle your private insurance company's idiosyncrasies and mixups with your husband's pension. And you have to do all of this on your own (my husband used to do this financial work).

As we remarked at the outset of this case illustration, federal and state governments have been loath to put a secure financial safety net under the ill and their families. The mixture of private, commercial, and public funding, as a support to family or individual funding, is the outcome. That combination can result, as is well known, in great depletion of family savings and considerable lowering of standards of living when the illness is severe and prolonged. Apparently, in many instances, impoverishment is at the end of the trail. As Mrs. Stutz's case illustrates vividly, the consequences also include collusion between government servants on the one side and professionals and caretakers on the other, as the latter seek to get public funding for their kin. Where the rules can be bent, disregarded, or cheated on, the knowledgeable may advise and assist the naive. Furthermore, citizens are socialized into new, suspicious attitudes toward their government insofar as its laws and its representatives are inconsiderate, even cruel. They are made increasingly aware—as is the general public, which is learning about this through the mass media as well as by word of mouth or by family experience—that something is wrong in the way this country provides for its desperately ill. Cases like that of Mrs. Stutz, as well as the visibility of Alzheimer's and AIDS in the media, are slowly but surely raising both moral and financial issues. At the same time, of course, the increasing costs of medicine and the tightening of the nation's budget are also part of the public awareness.

The ill and their families are trapped in a double predicament, part physical and part organizational or social. The government is perfectly capable of easing their financial burdens but does little in this regard. The dilemma must be faced not only by the families or for that matter by the federal and state governments, but also by the wider public. This becomes increasingly necessary with the increase in severely debilitating chronic illness.

Summary

Along with acute phases, deterioration is what the health care system is most concerned with, as are the practitioners who wish to prevent it or slow it down. What are the chief policy issues in this phase? For many of the chronically ill, particularly the elderly, savings have been drastically depleted by long illness. Other resources have also dwindled—adult children have moved away, friends have died or are also in fragile physical condition. They neither know about available services nor know how to find them, and would be ashamed anyhow to ask for them. Handling the Medicare billing adds to their anxiety and growing exhaustion. The likelihood of well spouses becoming ill also increases; this compounds their difficulties in maintaining their previous quality of life and mental health. People can also fall through the bureaucratic cracks because they do not officially qualify for services. In many cases, very little is actually necessary to ensure a longer life and maintain a desired quality of life. Other people, however, suffer from many difficulties and humiliations in dealing with government agencies. Health practitioners, lawyers, and the ill or caretakers may be forced into collusion by current government policies.

In these cases, we can see once again some of the consequences of the present policy of funding the ill and their caretakers. Federal and state governments have been reluctant to build a financial safety net under people who confront impoverishment because of catastrophic illnesses in the family. Thus these people are trapped in a predicament that has two aspects: one attributable to the illness itself, the other to the current health policies and their associated funding and organizational patterns. A health care system that does not conceive of the full range of these people's nonclinical problems as a multiple set of intersecting circumstances is in large measure ineffective.

The ill and their caretakers become extremely vulnerable

as physical condition as well as resources run downhill in tandem. Whatever stability of physical condition and of life has been attained is now threatened. The intervention of professionals or the offering of health services, even if this assistance is temporary, can contribute to restabilization and quality of life. Services that are inaccessible, services that require complicated or confusing "qualifications," and deficiencies in services actually available all contribute to the rate of decline, and to the number of people who will enter nursing homes rather than live out their remaining years or days at home.

THREE

$$* \; * \; * \; * \; *$$

Rethinking
Our Health Care System

In Part Three, we bring practice and policy together. The actual delivery of health care by practitioners is largely a reflection of policy issues and how they are faced at a more general level. At the same time, the larger policy issues should be derived from the practice of those who provide direct care and services to the chronically ill and their families, as well as from what the ill and their families need by way of services.

Chapter Ten outlines some general implications of our trajectory model for the perspectives and work of practitioners. They often suffer from professionalized viewpoints or organizational constraints; thinking of chronic illness as a trajectory can help practitioners work as partners with the ill and families in chronic illness management.

In Chapter Eleven, we present a number of policy implications of the fact that chronic illness is now the prevalent form of illness. We begin by summarizing how our perspective and its associated trajectory model differ from the views of other critics of the health care system, including those of the gerontological and rehabilitation experts whose views are perhaps closest to ours. We review what chronic illness might imply for a reconstitution of the American health system. We put home at the center of care and discuss in detail what this means. We talk about the intermeshing of care at home and the work of practitioners both in health facilities and when they visit the homes. We briefly address major policy issues—cost, technology, equity, bioethics, quality of life—in terms of chronic illness prevalence. We end with the need for new perspectives that will take the broader implications of chronic illness into account.

10

* * * * *

New Approaches
to Caring for
the Chronically Ill

In this chapter, we propose some practical and policy implications that can be derived from the case histories presented in earlier chapters. This chapter is not meant to give specific details on practice but rather to bring out relevant features of the trajectory model for the practitioner and to point out what policy changes are called for in order to put our suggestions into effect. The trajectory model is elaborated in our previous book (Corbin and Strauss, 1988).

This book has shown that the management of chronic illness is often approached in a very intellectual, professional, top-down manner, with a focus on the acute aspects of disease management. Without meaning to diminish the tremendous advances made in the delivery of health care within the last decade or the humanistic qualities of some of the more caring practitioners, we will briefly explain why health care delivery to the chronically ill and their families remains inadequate in many ways. A brief anecdote will help to illustrate what we mean.

As part of the requirements for a course on chronic illness, students were asked to write a paper on an aspect of its management. One student, a very caring nurse, turned in a paper about which she was most excited. In it, she argued that much of diabetic patients' noncompliance is due to the fact that they do not fully accept their disease. Hence, she proposed that compliance could be improved if clients were given counseling to help them accept their condition.

The student's concern with the emotional aspects of illness is admirable. Perhaps in some cases, nonadherence to regimens is related to nonacceptance of the disease. Yet there is something fundamentally wrong with her basic assumptions, though in many ways her thinking reflects that of health professionals at large. This is a top-down, one-sided view of the situation that fails to see what is really going on with patients and to see the problem from their perspective. Before jumping to the conclusion that a person is noncompliant it is necessary to ask: To what degree is a client following the regimen—not at all, in part, sometimes, all of the time? In trying to implement the regimen, what else does this person have to contend with? What is his or her life-style and how does the regimen fit with it? If the client is not following the regimen as prescribed, what is or is not being done and why? Moreover, what does it mean not to accept one's disease? Does not following a regimen necessarily indicate a lack of acceptance? Does it reflect the inability to integrate a regimen into the flow of one's daily life? The issue of compliance, though only one of the problems in chronic illness management, is a complicated one and quite illustrative of why a new way of thinking about illness, patients, and illness management is called for in the care of persons with chronic conditions.

When persons develop an acute illness, such as a noncomplicated infection, and are given regimens to follow, they know that after the course of therapy, they will probably be cured and can go on with their lives. It does not matter if the regimen causes some inconvenience, since after all it is only temporary. A chronic condition, however, means that people must live with symptoms and disabilities that must be managed for the rest of their lives. Furthermore, those lives must be *lived* despite illness. Integrating regimens into the flow of one's everyday life requires planning, thought, and working things out. We call this process the making of arrangements. For instance, a diabetic must arrange to eat, take insulin, and check urine or blood for glucose levels within a certain time or suffer consequences. Each of these tasks must somehow be integrated into the ongoing stream of daily activities. This requires making arrangements with oneself or others for the timing and content of meals, obtaining and maintaining equipment, and taking time out to perform the tasks.

Which of the following would be the more likely reason that busy executives or construction workers who have diabetes fail to follow a regimen as prescribed? (1) They don't accept their disease; (2) they don't know how to integrate the management of their condition with the normal tasks associated with working at a job where mealtimes, activity, schedules, intensity of work, and deadlines vary from day to day.

The most likely answer is the second. It is easy to be too busy, to forget, to find it inappropriate or embarrassing to stop what one is doing to inject oneself or eat. In such cases, flexibility in the job and the regimen is called for. Yet very few clients have the medical background to know how to achieve a balance between controlling their condition and doing their job. It takes considerable medical sophistication and experience with illness management to understand the subtleties of how illness affects you, where you can give and where you cannot. It is in making arrangements to handle problematic situations—carrying out regimens, finding resources, doing caretaking, and so forth— that the ill and their families need assistance. Yet it is in this very area that health professionals are most likely to fail in providing help.

There are two major reasons for this failure. One reason is that sometimes health professionals overlook or misidentify the important problems facing the chronically ill because of all the reasons outlined in this book. The other reason is not so simple. Very often practitioners see the problems and want to do something about them, but are constrained by the organizational conditions under which they work. One such condition is the necessity of giving priority to medical work involving great numbers of highly acute patients. This leaves little time or energy for what are considered nonmedical tasks like teaching or counseling. Agencies are paid only for the performance of "traditional medical tasks," which are probably sufficient when dealing with acute curable conditions, but not when dealing with chronic ones.

From a practitioner's standpoint, the management of chronic conditions is complicated. While the ideal can never be fully realized within society as it exists today, there is still much that can be done. Improving the delivery of health care by practitioners requires a knowledge base and a theoretical orientation, grounded in an understanding of the problems of managing chronic conditions and their impact. Though more and more knowledge is being developed in this area, there is still a considerable gap between knowledge and practice.

In Chapter Five of this book, we presented the trajectory framework. By thinking in terms of this framework, practitioners can combine empathy, knowledge, and skill to provide care designed to meet the special needs of the chronically ill and their families. Without repeating all that was said in that chapter, we can emphasize the following points.

First, chronic illness management must be seen through the eyes of those who are experiencing it. This requires health practitioners to take the role of the ill to see the problem or situation from their perspective. By putting oneself in the other's position, one has a better understanding of what it means to have an illness, symptoms, and disabilities that must be lived with and managed, and the living conditions under which one is trying to manage them. Thereby, one makes oneself sensitive to the types of arrangements that are needed to handle disabilities or to incorporate regimens into the context of daily living. An effective way of taking the role of the other is to ask oneself, how would I feel if I were in this situation? What would I need to manage under these conditions? What type of care would I want for myself or my family?

Second, chronic illness must be thought about as a lifelong course that passes through many phases, with the acute phase being only one of many. Thinking of chronic illness as a course enables practitioners to take into consideration the phases that came before and to plan for future ones, thus providing what is implied by the term *continuity of care.* The need to view the broad picture applies just as much to the nurses, physicians, and social workers who work in the intensive care unit as to those who work with clients out in the community.

Third, practitioners must not only think in terms of medical work but consider the biographical, spiritual, and everyday needs of the chronically ill and their families. This means that they have to ask questions about life-styles, about what each family member considers relevant aspects of self, what parts of self can be let go and what parts must be retained in order to maintain some sense of identity. On the basis of this information, practitioners can help families to make the arrangements that are important to them for carrying out medical, biographical, and everyday life work. Because arrangements are the key to successful management, they must be made with care, maintained, and remade in accordance with changes in illness phase, biography, or everyday life. Therefore, one of the first tasks of a practitioner working with the chronically ill and their families is to assess these arrangements. What arrangements are presently in effect? Where are they working? Where are they not? What kinds of resources are available? What else is needed?

Fourth, practitioners must develop collaborative partnerships with the ill and families in the management of chronic illness. Persons with chronic conditions usually have many years of experience and know how their bodies respond. They often know better than practitioners what works for them to relieve symptoms and what does not. They also know their life-styles and what changes in them are acceptable. If practitioners work with the ill and their families to develop the arrangements necessary to integrate illness and its management into their lives, there is a greater likelihood that the ill will follow through with regimens and other illness-related work. After all, the ill and their families are invested in seeing that life goes on. Those persons in special need of assistance from practitioners are the newly diagnosed or those with sudden changes in their illness course, biography, or everyday living.

Fifth, continued lifelong support is essential for the management of chronic conditions, though the type, amount, and intensity can vary with illness phase. During a crisis and immediately following hospitalization, a full complement of services may be needed. During more stable phases, an occasional telephone call or visit to assess conditions and demonstrate concern may suffice. Practitioners often feel that they have to intervene, to "do something"; otherwise they are not needed or not being effective (this is a holdover from an acute care perspective). Yet sometimes, all the chronically ill need is to know that there is someone to whom they can turn or somewhere to go should assistance be necessary.

Sixth, practitioners working with the chronically ill have to learn to "plant seeds" and wait for them to grow. People have to be taken where they are. Often they are not ready for arrangements that practitioners think should be undertaken, like using a lift to move someone in and out of bed, getting outside help, or placing someone in a nursing home. All one can do is make the suggestion and wait for the person to show readiness to do something about it.

Seventh, in severe debilitating illness and in ongoing illness, an "arrangements coordinator" or articulator of care is needed. People often do not know what services are available, how to obtain and use them, when they are needed, or what to do when the situation changes. Often, too, they are so overwhelmed by the illness and the work that they cannot evaluate the situation objectively. Nurses, social workers, and others who have a long-term professional relationship with ill persons and families can fill this role.

Finally, working with the chronically ill requires creativity, an ability to make do with what is at hand, and a vision of what can be done.

Before pointing out the organizational and national policy changes that are necessary in order for practitioners to carry out the mandates specified above, we would like to step back for a moment and discuss the importance of applying theoretical frameworks to practice. We have mentioned that the acute care model, while very relevant for the management of curable illnesses, fails to provide the direction needed for the management of chronic conditions. But to take this away leaves practitioners with nothing to guide their practice.

Working with the chronically ill in the manner we suggest

requires sensitivity, understanding, commitment, perseverance, and a strong knowledge base about chronic illness and the work necessary to manage it and its impact. In addition, it requires the ability to critically analyze people and situations. Furthermore, we realize that continued investment in persons and their problems can quickly lead to professional burnout and, in some cases, "going native"—that is, becoming so emotionally involved with the problems of a person or family that it becomes impossible to make rational judgments and to be effective in the professional role. Practitioners need frameworks to replace the medical model and they need frameworks that are pertinent to chronicity.

One such framework is the trajectory framework. It is grounded in studies of chronic illness management; therefore, it fits the management of chronicity more readily than the acute care model it replaces. It directs practitioners to be sensitive to the medical, biographical, and everyday needs and life-styles of those with chronic conditions and their families. At the same time, it allows them to use a rational and systematic approach to assess and analyze situations. It does not at all discount the medical aspect of management but rather adds to it the complex relationships between it and biographical and everyday aspects of people's lives. Using the trajectory framework enables practitioners to keep a balance between involvement and professional distance, between the medical and psychosocial, thereby forestalling or preventing consequences like burnout, going native, and appearing uncaring or not understanding.

A number of policy changes are necessary to put a framework such as this one into practice. The first is specialized training for practitioners that sensitizes them to the special needs and problems of the chronically ill. The second is a restructuring of the organization of hospitals, clinics, and other agencies from a strictly acute care focus to one that includes chronic care. This will increase flexibility in the types of services that are offered and in the allocation of staff and time for treating, teaching, and counseling the chronically ill and their families. Third is a decrease in the bureaucratic barriers to obtaining services and an organization of services according to trajectory phasing rather than by specific disease, so that they are more readily available to the ill, their families, and practitioners when they are needed, regardless of type of disease. Rehabilitation services within an institution should be just as available to the cancer patient as to the cardiac patient; likewise, hospice services should be available to each. Fourth is the provision of more grass-roots health care providers, like nurse practitioners, therapists, and counselors. These providers should work together and be located in the community and on the streets to provide direct care to clients and families, and to interface between clients and the larger health care delivery system.

There must be a grounded approach to policy-making regarding chronic illness. For practitioners, this begins with studying the problems of the chronically ill and their families, then developing frameworks that aid in determining what services are necessary to manage these problems. From there, the approach furthers the next step of moving to the policy-making arena, where relevant issues can be debated and policy made, thus leading us back full circle to the ill.

11

$* * * * *$

A Model for
Reorganizing
Health Care Delivery

Our reason for writing this book is to affect current perspectives on health care policy and practice. We have argued for and illustrated the vital importance of taking seriously the fact that most ill people are sick from a chronic illness. Chronic illness is, after all, the prevalent form of illness today. In the early chapters, we summarized major characteristics of these illnesses and presented some material on and frequent criticisms about health care policy, including Medicare and Medicaid. We noted that the health arena is large, rapidly changing, and full of conflict. We acknowledged that the criticisms made by people who are concerned with long-term care (principally experts in gerontology, rehabilitation, and long-term care) are closest to our own doubts about the American care system in general. These critics emphasize, particularly with regard to long-term care, failures in health policy and care—especially failures in continuity, flexibility, and responsiveness to and respectfulness of the ill themselves. The cases presented in Chapters Six through Nine provide vivid illustrations of precisely this kind of criticism.

As Vladeck (1983, p. 7) has said, this kind of criticism is "hardly radical or unfamiliar to [long-term] health care professionals." What, then, do we have to offer besides dotting the *i*'s and crossing the *t*'s? In Chapter Four, when analyzing some of the views of these professionals, we asserted that because these people are professionally trained and experienced as professionals, they see policy and practice largely from professionalized perspectives. These are somewhat intellectualized, they are often focused sharply on the present, and they generally take a top-down (an administrator's or practitioner's) rather than a grass-roots (an ill person's) perspective.

These critics think of failures in health care almost wholly in terms of long-term care. That is all to the good, but it tends to blur the complex relationships between acute and long-term care, as well as between the acute and nonacute statuses of the ill as they pass from one phase of illness to another. The critics' attack on the acute care perspective also diverts them from paying more attention to the relationships of the several phases of long-term illness. Indeed, they lack a clear and overarching conceptual framework for thinking about the total arc of work (Strauss, Fagerhaugh, Suczek, and Wiener, 1985) that is necessary for simultaneously managing a severe chronic illness and achieving as high a quality of life as possible.

The raison d'etre of this book is to supply that conceptualization and to argue for its usefulness. To that end, we have presented a view that is firmly grounded in what living with and managing illness looks like to those suffering from severe chronic illnesses. The ill have to think (whether constantly, frequently, or occasionally) in terms of their symptoms and disabilities as these pass through various phases, where each phase involves a process of adjusting to the illness and making or juggling decisions in relation to it.

The concept of trajectory captures those phenomena, both in general and in detail. This concept and its associated theoretical model, presented in Chapter Five, provide a background for our policy commentaries in later chapters as well as the discussion of practical implications in Chapter Ten. The model encompasses the entire course of illness—including all of the emergent phases—and, furthermore, relates the acute phases to the others.

In this chapter (a revised and expanded version of Strauss,

1987), we need to draw policy implications from this trajectory model. We suggest some that call for a radical shift of focus, organization, and resource flow in the health care system. The model builds on the points developed earlier. The most important points are these:

- A chronic illness *persists* over a lifetime.
- When severe, it may have *many* phases.
- Hospitals mainly care for the ill during the *acute* (and sometimes the dying) phases.
- Periodic visits to clinics and doctors' offices are mainly for *stabilizing* the illness or slowing its deterioration.
- During *all* but the acute phases, it is the ill and their families who do the major work of managing the illness.
- Therefore, the *home* should be at the very center of care. *All* other facilities and services should be oriented toward supplementing and facilitating the work done at home.
- In this altered division of labor, practitioners would continue to play vital and often crucial roles. Therefore, the *two* sides of the division of labor should be as sensibly and tightly *linked* as possible.

The last two points are of equal importance. Taken together, they imply an overall policy model that involves both care at home and care at health facilities.

Home care implies that we view this site as *the* center of care: along with, second, the provision of resources in the form of money, education, and support services. Then, third, that there be those in sufficient quantities and with sufficient quality to enhance and augment home care management; *and* (a very important ''and'') fourth, during *all* phases of every long-term illness.

Home care has several components. There is illness work to be done on a daily, and sometimes hourly, basis. There is the discovery, use, maintenance, and replenishing of resources in sufficient quantity and of adequate quality to get that work done in every phase of illness. There are essential work arrangements, without which the work could not be done. This illness work must be connected with other domestic work and with regard to considerations of personal identity.

Finally, and most important, all of this work at home should be conceptualized as ongoing. It goes on daily; it goes on forever—as long as the illness itself. For the practitioners, whether they visit the ill at home or the ill visit them at health facilities, this means that their interventions must fit into and be coordinated with the ongoing work of managing illness and disability in this context of daily life. Furthermore, these interventions, whether clinical or nonclinical, must be incorporated by the ill themselves into what is, after all, their work process.

Consider briefly what this means for the practitioners' standard term, *services,* and for their much-used injunction that "services should match needs." In the context of a client's overall trajectory, services as a concept can only mean that there is a division of labor in the entire work process. The ill and their intimates and caretakers do certain aspects of the work; the practitioners do other aspects. Sometimes their work overlaps. The services that practitioners offer or sell to the ill come down to resources and work arrangements that they bring to the total flow of illness work. These resources and arrangements supplement or substitute for existing ones. Matching needs with services means providing the right resources or instituting or supporting arrangements that are appropriate to the ongoing work flow as it streams through various phases of illness work and living. Viewing services and needs in this temporal context eliminates the somewhat static and present-oriented focus that often creeps into health care and health policy.

What we are advocating is not merely a building out to the home from current health facilities and agencies. Rather, we advocate their reconstitution in relation to a much more effective and badly needed home management. This requires greatly increasing the flow of resources to the home (where right now the caretakers are predominantly mothers and wives). This reconstitution of health facilities and agencies entails training practitioners to work more fully and sensitively with the ill, recognizing that the latter are true partners in working at their own care. We also need new kinds of facilities to take over, whether temporarily or permanently, when families can no longer give good care or manage their own lives in the face of any ill member's severe deterioration or dying.

The American health care system is, in effect, mainly in the business of funding and providing acute care; the bulk of illness management at home concerns other phases of illness, which constitute most of the ill person's life. Management at home, though not as medically complicated as management done in hospitals or clinics, is certainly as complicated in other ways. This is because of the complexity of the home context in which home management takes place, and the lifelong nature of the enterprise.

If stability is the most desirable physical condition in a chronic illness, then we must necessarily think of the work that must be engaged in to maintain a stable condition. Much of that work is nonclinical; yet it is usually linked, in complicated personal and interactional ways, with the more strictly medical aspects of care. Practitioners at health facilities are skilled at managing illnesses when they are acute. They are skilled too at bringing about stability when someone is acutely ill, and at suggesting to the patient the best methods (regimens) for increasing the probability of remaining stable. Practitioners are equally skilled, for precisely the same reasons, at increasing the probability of a comeback from an acute phase as well as shortening the period of comeback before a stable level is reached. However, it is not usual for physicians, nor perhaps for most nurses, to be formally trained in giving information and counsel to patients and kin concerning the social, psychological, and interactional aspects of chronic illness. Nor are they trained to transmit information and counsel that they have heard from some of their patients to others. Yet this is exactly what happens in self-help groups, and is part of the philosophies of some of those groups.

The professionals are indeed useful for slowing down and even to some extent blocking deterioration in the chronically ill, as well as increasing the probability of long periods of stability before the next drop in physical functioning. What other means can be added to the physician's armamentarium in this regard?

Obviously, many of the suggestions made by people who are concerned with the health of the elderly are part of the answer to that question. Yet it pays to think of the deterioration-stability relationship not merely in terms of the elderly but also in terms of young people in different phases of illness. If one considers the illness profiles of sufferers from severe arthritis at all ages, it will be apparent that all illness phases are represented except perhaps the dying, though there may be fear of dying too. Diabetes is another instance, although the typical diabetic profiles are considerably different from the arthritic ones.

     If it is true that the central drama of illness management takes place in the home, then the central actor on stage is certainly the ill person. He or she is often joined by an intimate who not only shares the work but is indispensable to it. If the ill person is exceedingly ill, as with severe stroke or Alzheimer's disease, the intimate may do almost all of the work, the ill person sharing little of it. Our other research on chronic illness has shown us that the patient in a hospital also does a great deal of work, some of it visible and some not, although it is essentially unrecognized by the hospital personnel (Strauss, Fagerhaugh, Suczek, and Wiener, 1982, 1985; Fagerhaugh, Strauss, Suczek, and Wiener, 1987). The work includes keeping one's body absolutely still during a procedure, negotiating for pain relief, and monitoring the staff's work for competence and safety. Much of how the patient carries out the work is based on knowledge gained from years of managing his or her illness. After leaving the hospital, the ill person—no longer "a patient" but a responsible person—continues with management work. Most of this is true for the spouse or other intimates as well.

     Since the ill person is the central actor all through this lifelong plot line, why not take his or her role seriously? By seriously, we mean in an organizational or programmatic sense. Today, the patient's central work role is ignored or even bemoaned because of patients' frequent "irresponsibility." This accusation is reflected in the considerable literature on "noncompliance." Well-intentioned but secondary efforts at teaching patients and kin shortly before discharge from hospital are steps in the right direction, but they do not meet today's situation

head-on. Indeed, the teaching is mainly focused on the do's and
don't's of the regimen, not on the conditions that might help
or hinder carrying out the regimen and controlling the symptoms, nor on how to monitor signs of clinical danger in relatively
sophisticated ways.

Perhaps the most explicit recognition of the patient as an
essential member of the health team is in the case of cardiac
and other organ transplant patients. If one does not teach and
counsel them and their spouses, and of course monitor the work
they do at home, those patients will surely increase one's mortality statistics. Yet a recent compendium of review articles by
experts on cardiac transplantation actually devoted only one
slender chapter to psychosocial aspects, and the information
given was, by generally accepted standards of social science,
rudimentary and unsatisfactory (Evans and others, 1985). Even
the voices of transplant patients and kin are heard only faintly.
Still, that situation is better than with our own interviewees,
whose voices are almost wholly unheard by practitioners and
policymakers, or if heard, then unnoted. The same is true, apparently, of a considerable proportion of people who have written
about their own, their spouse's, or their children's illnesses.

We touch next on a central point in what some will undoubtedly think is an impossibly idealistic set of policy suggestions. There will have to be an effective linkage of work done
at home and work done in the health facilities. The problems
of implementation would, of course, be enormous, since our
health care system is not at all organized in those terms: not
the facilities, not the training, not the basic perspectives of practitioners. But these problems have to be faced, given the implications of chronic illness prevalence. Staffs in health facilities
must think in terms of chronic illness trajectories. When patients are hospitalized, they should be viewed as now in an acute
phase that either was preceded by other phases (which should
be discovered and taken into account) or is itself the first phase
(which is very different from a repeated acute phase). Staff should
take seriously also the implications that they are seeing only
cross-sections of a trajectory that will extend far beyond the small
slice of time that the patient spends at the facility. The implica-

tions of this view for care at health facilities, and for training that would fit this, are obviously far-reaching. It is true that such change is actually coming, although slowly, since even on ICUs personnel are increasingly concerned with rehabilitative work in terms of patients' recovery after hospitalization. On pediatric cardiac units, too, staffs are sometimes keenly aware of the necessity of working with parents before a child is sent home (Smith, 1985); alas, this is not characteristic of what happens on intensive care nurseries. One can also see changes in decreasing isolation of hospitals from homes in the increased development of hospital outreach programs, although these are still restricted almost wholly to the immediate recovery period. Rehabilitation services are still not much oriented to the chronically ill; this is another area where radical change is needed. However, rather than give a laundry list of specific suggestions about health facility–home articulation, we shall only repeat that work in health facilities and work at home need to be much more tightly interwoven. Innovative programs in this regard would profit from thinking in terms of our trajectory model.

We turn next to more traditional policy concerns. We shall make only the most general, positional statements about them, since our aim is to give a basis for shifting policy perspectives on chronic illness, not to offer a detailed blueprint for policy change. The first issue is funding. What is needed is a general reconsideration of—and widespread public debate about—why the overwhelming proportion of public funding goes for facilities, training, research, and practice that are so narrowly focused on the acute and immediate recovery phases of Americans' long-term, lifelong illnesses. There is, of course, the continued rising cost of health care, but this is probably linked with the essentially medical or clinical care given during acute phases of chronic illness. Nobody yet knows whether shifting funds toward home care would stop or slow down the inflation of costs, but at least the money might be more effectively spent. When cost-cutting policies, such as those that have dominated recent governmental regulations, are considered in the future, questions might well be asked about what the effect of new measures will be on the deterioration or stability of patients discharged from disproportionately costly hospital care, and whether the new measures might not actually add to the costs of containing illness.

We agree with long-term care critics of the health care system that there should be a redirection of funding toward home care; also toward the improvement of nursing homes, especially through staffing them with genuinely trained and psychologically sensitive nursing personnel. Not only should actual services be funded; appropriate financial mechanisms can be instituted for giving exhausted spouses and caretakers periods of respite and for keeping the greatly deteriorated ill out of nursing homes by minimal financial support of them or their families. Financial support is also needed for training the health workers who visit homes in the kinds of considerations raised in Chapter Ten, so that they will understand better how to give appropriate home care.

Another prominent issue debated in the health arena is that of equity, or equal opportunity for access to health care services. Advocacy of equity is deeply rooted in a humanitarian reform tradition that goes back many decades. Much as we subscribe to the demand for equity, we believe that its proponents are much too focused on access to acute care. They will say, perhaps, "first things first." Our answer to that argument is that demands for equity should be updated to include equitable and appropriate care for phases of lifelong illness. Even if health facilities were to become completely accessible, it would hardly solve the health problems of poorer Americans. As we have seen, even the working-class ill who have fair access to facilities and coverage for medical expenses need much more by way of diverse services and supportive arrangements. The impoverished have more chronic illnesses and are sicker from them, die earlier from them, and quite obviously need more than acute care services. The same can be said for the many American ethnic groups, each of which has different cultural traditions that sometimes affect the services they need and how they should be offered. For such cultural reasons, some ethnic groups find the health services less accessible than they should be. This is part of the equity problem, too. The traditional views of equity, in short, need some rethinking.

The same is true of another issue, that of bioethics. The debate that has arisen about medicine in relation to questions of morality has been focused on medical high technology and its impact on a single phase of illness, that of dying. If we think in terms of chronic illness, ethical considerations are really associated with each of its several phases. For instance, should the ill be told about all of the potential side effects of cancer therapy, or only some? When? How? By whom? Our case illustrations in earlier chapters suggest other bioethical questions: Should the ill and their families become impoverished before Medicaid support begins? Should physicians inform their patients fully and carefully of potential major side effects of technologies and surgeries before utilizing them?

Another important issue related to medical technology is that the unceasing debate over technological assessment is confined essentially to cost and safety issues of technology that is in the service of acute care. Thinking in terms of chronic illness would enlarge greatly the sphere of innovation for people who are in other phases of illness—much as, in recent years, the disabled have profited from relatively simple but wonderfully effective new inventions like walkers and electrified wheelchairs. Only now are we beginning to get devices and tests that allow self-monitoring at home of blood pressure and of diabetic signs. There should be concerted attempts to develop and improve such low-cost technologies for home use and funding for the necessary research and training of the ill.

In closing this book, we would like to note an assumption that lies behind our central argument. Whereas for infectious disease, the aim of medicine is to save people, or in less extreme illnesses, to get them well more quickly. For chronic illness, however, the clinical aim must necessarily be something else. Even if survival or delaying death is the immediate aim, nevertheless once the patient is out of danger then clinical effort can only slow down deterioration or mitigate or relieve symptoms. This means an improved quality of life because of fewer restrictions on what the body can do and therefore on what activities can be engaged in, accomplished, or enjoyed. Improving the quality of life is what the health practitioners are really in the business of doing—as are the ill and their families. This, too, is what the health policymakers should strive to contribute toward. An undue medical-clinical focus, and a narrow focus on acute illness at that, is both a betrayal of what modern medicine is capable of contributing to and a betrayal of public trust in the health professions.

We realize, of course, how difficult it is to make any major change in the nation's approach to illness, considering the financial and other problems that it faces, the diverse political stances, and the length of time it takes for any large-scale change to occur. Right now seems the most hopeless of times for advocating such views—for right now, families are being brutally forced by the cutbacks in hospitals and agencies to shoulder more and more of the burdens of their own care. Nevertheless, it is our hope that if enough people say the same thing for a long enough time, those with the power to make a difference will hear the message and begin to institute the necessary reforms. The inexorable impact of an aging population should certainly hasten that day.

To be chronically ill in America is not just to be an individual struggling against fate; it is to be in a societal condition shared by all of the chronically ill. No industrial country seems to have solved the psychological and social problems attending and affecting their physical plight by instituting and maintaining even approximately effective and humane organizational arrangements. This country certainly has not done so. One of our national dilemmas rests on the propensity to further, extol, and even glorify individualism, on the one hand; and on the other hand to yield with seeming reluctance to collective action and governmental implementation, while really pursuing these with vigor and receiving their benefits willingly. These contradictions have entered into the nation's handling of the chronically ill. Characteristically, our technologically and organizationally oriented society has better confronted chronic illness itself than issues concerning the chronically ill, letting the ill more or less fend for themselves as responsible individuals and citizens. This forces the ill to be the centrally responsible agents in their own care—rather than recognizing that in reality they are the central workers who are abetted by health practitioners. This policy strategy fails to face up to the far-reaching implications of chronic illness prevalence, and it prevents us from more fully meeting the responsibilities of a genuinely humane society.

In this book we have attempted to build a theoretical framework for the management of chronic illness, and thus to lay the groundwork for policy planners to reason in somewhat different terms than they now do. They need this kind of theoretical and empirical foundation in order to build health policy more realistically. This includes building it in terms of what both the ill and their families and the health professionals can do together. Such an empirically grounded theoretical approach can help toward achieving an equitable and effective balance between societal and individual considerations.

Vladeck and Firman have come close to our position, though without offering such a specific model as the trajectory one. They write: "Reorientation of the health care system to respond better to the problems of the chronically ill is thus one of the central challenges for medicine in the coming decades, but one that poses formidable problems, since it involves fundamental changes not only in the financing and organization of formal services, but also in the definition of roles for various groups of professional and nonprofessional personnel, the attenuation of boundaries between the medical and nonmedical spheres, and a rethinking of the balance between technical and samaritan components of medical service. . . . Such programs cannot be peripheral appendages to the existing system; they must become the existing system. . . . Development of effective and affordable systems of chronic care as the core of the health care system is the central task for health policy in the coming decades" (Vladeck and Firman, 1983, pp. 142, 148).

Our book has focused on the need of such a chronic illness perspective for an effective health policy. Throughout, however, we have implicitly referred to the implications of chronic illness prevalence for society at large. These broader implications need to be studied and understood before major changes in policy will become politically possible. Here are a few obvious impacts on industrialized nations of chronic illness: the rise of health care as a major industry; the increasing proportion of the gross national product that health care consumes; the primary developments in the structure of health facilities and health occupations; the crosscutting of health issues with important social and ideological movements, such as patients' rights, the feminist movement, and the gay rights movement (especially in relation to the AIDS epidemic); various bioethical issues and debates over them; the increasingly prominent role of health or health-related news and human interest stories in the mass media; the widespread anxiety over environmental causes of chronic illnesses like cancer and heart diseases. Relevant also is the development of international concern—perhaps furor is a more apt description—over AIDS. AIDS is a deadly and dreadful infectious disease; but it is also a chronic illness for those who contract it and must live with it for some months or years before they die. The multiplicity of public, professional, and scientific issues that this illness has spawned is astonishing, and its impact on customs, institutions, and perspectives is only beginning. Not every chronic illness has that kind of major impact on the social fabric, but collectively they certainly do. This, too, should be part of a chronic illness perspective.

$$\text{\Huge ✳ ✳ ✳}$$

References

Anderson, O. *The American Health Services: A Growth Enterprise Since 1875.* Ann Arbor, Mich.: Health Administration Press, 1985.

Anderson, T. "Educational Frame of Reference: An Additional Model for Rehabilitation Medicine." *Archives of Physical Medicine and Rehabilitation,* 1978, *59,* 203–206.

Arling, G., and McAuley, W. "The Feasibility of Public Payments for Family Caregiving." *The Gerontologist,* 1983, *23,* 300–306.

Bauwens, E., Anderson, S., and Buergin, E. "Chronic Illness." In W. Phipps, B. Long, and N. Woods (eds.), *Medical Surgical Nursing.* St. Louis, Mo.: Mosby, 1983.

Bazanger, I. "Les Maladies Chroniques et leur Ordre Negocié" [The chronic illnesses and their negotiated order]. *Revue Française de Sociologie,* 1986, *27,* 3–27.

Becker, G., and Kaufman, S. "Old Age, Rehabilitation and Research: A Review of the Issues." Unpublished paper, Department of Social and Behavioral Sciences, University of California, San Francisco, 1987.

Becker, H., Geer, B., Hughes, E., and Strauss, A. *Boys in White.* Chicago: University of Chicago Press, 1964.

Becker, M., and Maiman, I. "Sociobehavioral Determinants of Compliance with Health and Medical Care Recommendations." *Medical Care,* 1975, *13,* 10–24.

Bowe, E. *Handicapping People.* New York: Harper & Row, 1978.

Brody, E. " 'Women in the Middle' and Family Help to Older People." *The Gerontologist,* 1981, *21,* 471–480.

Brody, S. "Strategic Planning: The Catastrophic Approach."
The Gerontologist, 1987, *27,* 131–138.

Brody, S., Poulshock, S., and Masciocchi, C. "The Family
Caring Unit: A Major Consideration in the Long-Term Care
Support System." *The Gerontologist,* 1978, *18,* 555–561.

Bucher, R., and Stelling, J. *Becoming Professional.* Newbury Park,
Calif.: Sage, 1977.

Budrys, G. *Planning the Nation's Health.* New York: Greenwood,
1986.

Bury, M. "Illness as Biographical Disruption." *Sociology of Health
and Illness,* 1982, *4,* 167–182.

Butler, L., and Newacheck, P. "Health and Social Factors Affecting Long-Term Care Policy." In J. Meltzer, F. Farrow,
and H. Richman (eds.), *Policy Options and Long-Term Care.*
Chicago: University of Chicago Press, 1981.

Butler, R. "Nursing Home Care: An Impossible Situation
Unless." *International Journal of Aging and Human Development,*
1977–1978, *39,* 73–76.

Charmaz, K. "Loss of Self: A Fundamental Form of Suffering
in the Chronically Ill." *Sociology of Health and Illness,* 1983,
5, 168–195.

Charmaz, K. "Struggling for a Self: Identity Levels of the
Chronically Ill." In J. Roth and P. Conrad (eds.), *Research
in the Sociology of Health Care.* Vol. 6: *The Experience and Management of Chronic Illness.* Greenwich, Conn.: JAI Press, 1987.

Childress, J. "Sociocultural Metaphors." In H. Schwartz (ed.),
Dominant Issues in Medical Sociology. (2nd ed.) New York: Random House, 1987.

Cluff, L. "Chronic Disease, Function and the Quality of Care."
Social Science and Medicine, 1981, *34,* 299–304.

Cole, S., O'Conner, S., and Bennett, L. "Self-Help Groups
for Clinic Patients with Chronic Illness." *Primary Care,* 1979,
6, 325–340.

Coleman, V., Summers, T., and Leonard, F. "Till Death Do Us
Part: Caregiving Wives of Severely Disabled Husbands." Gray
Paper no. 7. Washington, D.C.: Older Women's League,
1982.

Conrad, P. "The Meaning of Medication: Another Look at
Compliance." *Social Science and Medicine,* 1985, *20,* 29–37.

Conrad, P. "The Experience of Illness: Recent and New Directions." In J. Roth and P. Conrad (eds.), *Research in the Sociology of Health Care.* Vol. 6: *The Experience and Management of Chronic Illness.* Greenwich, Conn.: JAI Press, 1987.

Corbin, J., and Strauss, A. "Issues Concerning Regimen Managing in the Home." *Ageing and Society,* 1985, *5,* 249–265.

Corbin, J., and Strauss, A. *Unending Work and Care: Managing Chronic Illness at Home.* San Francisco: Jossey-Bass, 1988.

Crossman, L., London, C., and Barry, C. "Older Women Caring for Disabled Spouses: A Model for Supportive Services." *The Gerontologist,* 1981, *21,* 464–470.

Curtin, M., and Lubkin, I. "What Is Chronicity?" In I. Lubkin (ed.), *Chronic Illness: Impact and Interventions.* Boston: Jones and Barlett, 1986.

Davis, K., and Rowland, D. "Uninsured and Underserved: Inequities in Health Care in the United States." In H. Schwartz (ed.), *Dominant Issues in Medical Sociology.* (2nd ed.) New York: Random House, 1983.

Davis, M. *Living with Multiple Sclerosis.* Springfield, Ill.: Thomas, 1973.

Dawson, D., and Adams, P. "Current Estimates from the National Interview Survey, United States, 1986." In U.S. Public Health Service, *Vital and Health Statistics.* Series 10, no. 164, Department of Health and Human Services publication (*PHS*). Washington D.C.: U.S. Government Printing Office, 1987.

De Mille, A. *Reprieve: A Memoir.* Garden City, N.Y.: Doubleday, 1981.

Denzin, N. *The Recovering Alcoholic.* Newbury Park, Calif: Sage, 1986.

Dewey, J. *Art as Experience.* New York: Balach, 1934.

Dunphy, J. "For the Elderly, No Place Like Home." *Detroit Free Press,* May 15, 1984, pp. 1b, 3b.

Estes, C., and Lee, P. "Health Problems and Policy Issues of Old Age." In L. Aiken and D. Mechanic (eds.), *Applications of Social Science to Clinical Medicine and Health Policy.* New Brunswick, N.J.: Rutgers University Press, 1986.

Evans, R., and others (eds.). *The National Heart Transplant Study: A Final Report.* Seattle, Wash.: Battelle Human Affairs Research Center, 1985.

Fagerhaugh, S., and Strauss, A. *The Politics of Pain Management: Staff-Patient Interaction.* Reading, Mass: Atherton, 1977.

Fagerhaugh, S., Strauss, A., Suczek, B., and Wiener, C. *Hazards in Hospital Care: Ensuring Patient Safety.* San Francisco: Jossey-Bass, 1987.

Feder, J. "Effects of Changing Federal Health Policies on the General Public, the Aged and the Disabled." *Bulletin of the New York Academy of Medicine,* 1983, *59,* 41–49.

Fein, R. (ed.). *Health Planning in the United States.* Vol. 1. Washington, D.C.: National Academy Press, 1981.

Fein, R. *Medical Care, Medical Costs: The Search for a Health Insurance Policy.* Cambridge, Mass.: Harvard University Press, 1986.

Feldman, D. "Chronic Disabling Illness: A Holistic View." *Journal of Chronic Disease,* 1974, *27,* 287–291.

Fengler, A., and Goodrich, N. "Wives of Elderly Disabled Men: The Hidden Patients." *The Gerontologist,* 1979, *19,* 175–183.

Fordyce, W. "A Behavioral Perspective in Rehabilitation." In G. Albrecht (ed.), *The Sociology of Physical Disability and Rehabilitation.* Pittsburgh, Pa.: University of Pittsburgh Press, 1976.

Fowler, W. "Viability of Physical Medicine and Rehabilitation in the 1980s." *Archives of Physical Medicine and Rehabilitation,* 1982, *63,* 1–5.

Freidson, E. *Profession of Medicine.* New York: Dodd, Mead, 1970a.

Freidson, E. *Professional Dominance.* Chicago: Aldine, 1970b.

Freidson, E. *Professional Powers.* Chicago: University of Chicago Press, 1986.

Friedemann, M-L. "The Agency Maze." In I. Lubkin (ed.), *Chronic Illness: Impact and Interventions.* Boston: Jones and Bartlett, 1986.

Gartner, A., and Riessman, F. (eds.). *The Self-Help Revolution.* New York: Human Services Press, 1984.

Gerhardt, U., and Brieskorn-Zinke, M. "The Normalization of Hemodialysis at Home." In J. Roth and S. Ruzek (eds.), *Research in the Sociology of Health Care.* Vol. 4: *The Adoption and Social Consequences of Medical Technologies.* Greenwich, Conn.: JAI Press, 1986.

Gerson, E., and Strauss, A. "Time for Living: Problems in Chronic Illness Care." *Social Policy*, 1975, *36*, 12–18.

Guillemin, J., and Holstrom, L. *Mixed Blessings: Intensive Care for Newborns.* New York: Oxford University Press, 1986.

Haldeman, S. *Modern Developments in the Principles and Practice of Chiropractic.* East Norwalk, Conn.: Appleton-Century-Crofts, 1980.

Harding, R., Heller, J., and Kesler, R. "The Critically Ill Child in the Primary Care Setting." *Primary Care*, 1979, *62*, 322–329.

Hooyman, N., Gonyea, J., and Montgomery, R. "The Impact of In-Home Services Termination on Family Caregivers." *The Gerontologist*, 1985, *25*, 141–145.

Hughes, E. "Professions." In E. Hughes, *The Sociological Eye.* Vol. 2. Chicago: Aldine-Atherton, 1971.

Jillings, C. "Is Chronic Illness a Relevant Topic for the Critical Care Nurse?" *Critical Care Nurse*, 1987, *7*, 14–17.

Kaslof, L. (ed.). *Wholistic Dimensions of Healing: Resource Guide.* Garden City, N.Y.: Doubleday, 1978.

Kasper, J., Walden, D., and Wilensky, G. "Who Are the Uninsured?" *National Medical Care Expenditures Survey Data Preview,* no. 1. Hyattsville, Md.: National Center for Health Services Research, 1978.

Kaufman, C. "Rights and Provision of Health Care: A Comparison of Canada, Great Britain, and the United States." In H. Schwartz, *Dominant Issues in Medical Sociology.* (2nd ed.) New York: Random House, 1987.

Kaufman, S., and Becker, G. "Stroke: Health Care on the Periphery." *Social Science and Medicine*, 1986, *22*, 983–989.

Kottke, F. "The Focus of Rehabilitation Medicine." *Archives of Physical Medicine and Rehabilitation*, 1980, *61*, 1–6.

Kutner, N. "Social Worlds and Identity in End-Stage Renal Disease." In J. Roth and P. Conrad (eds.), *Research in the Sociology of Health Care.* Vol. 6: *The Experience and Management of Chronic Illness.* Greenwich, Conn.: JAI Press, 1987.

Labrie, V. "Lupus: Managing a Complex Chronic Disability." Unpublished doctoral dissertation, Department of Social and Behavioral Sciences, University of California, San Francisco, 1986.

La Porte, V., and Rubin, J. (eds.). *Reform and Regulation in Long-Term Care.* New York: Praeger, 1979.

La Vor, J. "Long-Term Care: A Challenge to Service Systems." In V. La Porte and J. Rubin (eds.), *Reform and Regulation in Long-Term Care.* New York: Praeger, 1979.

Lee, A. *Employment, Unemployment, and Health Insurance.* Cambridge, Mass.: Abt Books, 1979.

Lee, J., and Stein, M. "Eliminating Duplication in Home Care for the Elderly." *Health and Social Work,* 1980, *5,* 29–36.

Levy, N. "The Chronically Ill Patient." *Psychiatric Quarterly,* 1979, *51,* 189–197.

Lewin, E., and Olesen, O. *Women, Health, and Healing: A New Perspective.* New York: Tavistock-Methuen, 1985.

Locker, D. *Disability and Disadvantage: The Consequences of Chronic Illness.* New York: Tavistock, 1983.

Lubkin, I. (ed.). *Chronic Illness: Impact and Interventions.* Boston: Jones and Bartlett, 1986.

Mace, N., and Babins, P. *The 36-Hour Day.* Baltimore, Md.: Johns Hopkins University Press, 1981.

Maines, D. "Time and Biography in Diabetic Experience." *Mid-American Review of Sociology,* 1983, *8,* 103–117.

Maines, D. "The Social Arrangements of Diabetic Self-Help Groups." In A. Strauss and others, *Chronic Illness and the Quality of Life.* (2nd ed.) St. Louis, Mo.: Mosby, 1984.

Maretzki, T. "Including the Physician in Healer-Centered Research." In R. Hahn and A. Gaines (eds.), *Physicians of Western Medicine.* Doordrecht, The Netherlands: Reidel, 1985.

Massie, R., and Massie, S. *Journey.* New York: Knopf, 1973.

Mayo, L. *Problem and Challenge.* New York: National Health Council, 1956.

Mead, L. "Health Policy: The Need for Governance." *Annals,* 1977, pp. 39–57.

Mechanic, D. "A Brief Anatomy of the American Health Care System." In D. Mechanic (ed.), *From Advocacy to Allocation: The Evolving American Health Care System.* New York: Free Press, 1986.

Meltzer, J., Farrow, F., and Richman, H. (eds.). *Policy Options and Long-Term Care.* Chicago: University of Chicago Press, 1981.

Mizrahi, T. *Getting Rid of Patients: Contradictions in the Training of Internists.* New Brunswick, N.J.: Rutgers University Press, 1987.

Neifing, T. "Financial Impact." In I. Lubkin (ed.), *Chronic Illness: Impact and Interventions.* Boston: Jones and Bartlett, 1986.

Neuberger, G., and Woods, S. "Alternative Modalities." In I. Lubkin (ed.), *Chronic Illness: Impact and Interventions.* Boston: Jones and Bartlett, 1986.

Pear, R. "Protecting Family Assets: A New Breed of Medicaid Counselors Steps In." *New York Times,* Sept. 16, 1987, p. 12.

Reif, L. "Beyond Medical Intervention: Strategies for Managing Life in the Face of Chronic Illness." In M. Davis and others (eds.), *Nurses in Practice: A Perspective on Work Environments.* St. Louis, Mo.: Mosby, 1975a.

Reif, L. "Cardiacs and Normals: The Social Construction of a Disability." Unpublished doctoral dissertation, Department of Social and Behavioral Sciences, University of California, San Francisco, 1975b.

Relman, A. "The New Medical-Industrial Complex." In H. Schwartz (ed.), *Dominant Issues in Medical Sociology.* (2nd ed.) New York: Random House, 1987.

Rice, D., and Hodgson, T. "Social and Economic Implications in the United States." In U.S. Public Health Service, *Vital and Health Statistics.* Series 3, no. 20. Department of Health and Human Services publication no. PHS–81–1404. Washington, D.C.: U.S. Government Printing Office, 1981.

Rice, D. and La Plante, M. "The Burden of Multiple Chronic Conditions: Past Trends and Policy Implications." Paper presented at the annual meeting of the American Public Health Association, Las Vegas, Nevada, Oct. 1986.

Roth, J. "The Public Hospital: Refuge for Damaged Humans." In A. Strauss (ed.), *Where Medicine Fails.* (4th ed.) New Brunswick, N.J.: Transaction, 1984.

Roth, J., and Ruzek, S. (eds.). *Research in the Sociology of Health Care.* Vol. 4: *The Adoption and Social Consequences of Medical Technologies.* Greenwich, Conn.: JAI Press, 1986.

Rothberg, J. "The Rehabilitation Team: Future Direction." *Archives of Physical Medicine and Rehabilitation,* 1981, *62,* 407–410.

Sackett, D., and Haynes, R. (eds.). *Compliance with Therapeutic Regimens*. Baltimore, Md.: Johns Hopkins University Press, 1976.

Sackett, D., and Snow, J. "The Magnitude of Compliance and Noncompliance." In R. Haynes, D. Taylor, and D. Sackett (eds.), *Compliance in Health Care*. Baltimore, Md.: Johns Hopkins University Press, 1979.

Schank, A. "Rehabilitation." In I. Lubkin (ed.), *Chronic Illness: Impact and Interventions*. Boston: Jones and Bartlett, 1986.

Schneider, J., and Conrad, P. *Having Epilepsy: The Experience and Control of Illness*. Philadelphia: Temple University Press, 1983.

Schroeder, S., and Showstack, J. "The Dynamics of Medical Technology in Use: Analysis and Policy Options." In S. Altman and R. Blendon (eds.), *Medical Technology: The Culprit Behind Health Care Costs?* Washington, D.C.: U.S. Department of Health, Education and Welfare, 1979.

Schwartz, H. "Irrationality as a Feature of Health Care in the United States." In H. Schwartz (ed.), *Dominant Issues in Medical Sociology*. (2nd ed.) New York: Random House, 1987.

Scott, R. "Professionals in Hospitals: Technology and the Organization of Work." In B. Georgepoulos (ed.), *Organization Research on Health Institutions*. Ann Arbor: Institute for Social Research, University of Michigan Press, 1972.

Smith, A. "Mothers as Life Agent Strategists in Neonatal Intensive Care Nurseries." Unpublished doctoral dissertation, Department of Social and Behavioral Sciences, University of California, San Francisco, 1985.

Sontag, S. *Illness as Metaphor*. New York: Farrar, Straus & Giroux, 1979.

Speedling, E. *Heart Attack: The Family Response at Home and in the Hospital*. New York: Tavistock, 1982.

Strauss, A. "Health Policy and Chronic Illness." *Society*, 1987, *25*, 33–39.

Strauss, A., Fagerhaugh, S., Suczek, B., and Wiener, C. "The Work of Hospitalized Patients." *Social Science and Medicine*, 1982, *16*, 977–986.

Strauss, A., Fagerhaugh, S., Suczek, B., and Wiener, C. *The Social Organization of Medical Work*. Chicago: University of Chicago Press, 1985.

Strauss, A., and Glaser, B. *Chronic Illness and the Quality of Life.* St. Louis, Mo.: Mosby, 1975.

Strauss, A., and others. *Chronic Illness and the Quality of Life.* (2nd ed.) St. Louis, Mo.: Mosby, 1984.

Svarstad, B. "Physician-Patient Communication and Patient Conformity with Medical Advice." In D. Mechanic (ed.), *Growth of Bureaucratic Medicine.* New York: Wiley, 1976.

Thomas, L. *The Living Cell.* New York: Bantam Books, 1974.

U.S. General Accounting Office. *The Elderly Should Benefit from Expanded Home Health Care but Increasing These Services Will Not Insure Cost Reductions.* Washington, D.C.: U.S. Government Printing Office, 1982.

Vaisrub, S. *Medicine's Metaphors: Messages and Menaces.* Oradell, N.J.: Medical Economics, 1977.

Verville, R. "The Rehabilitation Amendments of 1978: What Do They Mean for Comprehensive Rehabilitation?" *Archives of Physical Medicine and Rehabilitation,* 1979, *60,* 141–144.

Vladeck, B. "Two Steps Forward, One Back: The Changing Agenda of Long-Term Home Care Reform." *Pride Institute Journal of Long-Term Home Care,* 1983, *2,* 1–7.

Vladeck, B. "Meeting the Needs of the Elderly: A Client-Based Approach." Paper presented at the Conference on Strategies, Services, Structures—Quality Care for the Elderly: Meeting the Financial Challenge, San Diego, Calif., Feb. 13, 1984.

Vladeck, B. "The Static Dynamics of Long-Term Health Policy." In M. Lewin (ed.), *The Health Policy Agenda.* Washington, D.C.: American Enterprise Institute, 1985.

Vladeck, B., and Firman, J. "The Aging of Population and Health Services." *Annals A.A.P.S.S.,* 1983, *1,* 132–148.

Waitzkin, H. "Community-Based Health Care: Contradictions and Challenges." *Annals of Internal Medicine,* 1983, *98,* 235–242.

Ware, J. "The Assessment of Health Status." In L. Aiken and D. Mechanic (eds.), *Applications of Social Science to Clinical Medicine and Health Policy.* New Brunswick, N.J.: Rutgers University Press, 1986.

Warren, V. "A Powerful Metaphor: Medicine as War." Unpublished paper, cited in H. Schwartz (ed.), *Dominant Issues in Medical Sociology.* (2nd ed.) New York: Random House, 1987.

Wheeler-Lachowycz, J. "How to Use Your VNA." *American Journal of Nursing,* 1983, *83,* 1164–1167.

Wiener, C., Fagerhaugh, S., Suczek, B., and Strauss, A. "Trajectories, Biographies and the Evolving Medical Technology Scene: Labor and Delivery and the Intensive Care Nursery." *Sociology of Health and Illness,* 1979, *1,* 261–283.

Wilensky, G., and Berk, M. "The Health Care of the Poor and the Role of Medicaid." *Health Affairs,* 1982, *1,* 93–100.

Winn, S., and McCaffree, K. "Issues Involved in the Development of a Prepaid Capitation Plan for Long-Term Care Services." *The Gerontologist,* 1979, *19,* 184–190.

Wolpe, P. "The Maintenance of Professional Authority: Acupuncture and the American Physician." *Social Problems,* 1985, *32,* 409–424.

Woods, C., and Neuberger, G. "Alternative Modalities." In I. Lubkin (ed.), *Chronic Illness: Impact and Interventions.* Boston: Jones and Bartlett, 1986.

Zola, I. "Structural Constraints in the Doctor-Patient Relationships: The Case of Non-Compliance." In L. Eisenberg and A. Kleinman (eds.), *the Relevance of Social Science for Medicine.* Dordrecht, The Netherlands: Reidel, 1981.

Zola, I. *Missing Pieces: A Chronicle of Living with a Disability.* Philadelphia: Temple University Press, 1982.

$$\ast\ast\ast$$

Index